Dictionary of Eye Care and Vision Science

Technical terminology in eye care and vision sciences can be challenging to navigate, particularly in busy clinical and academic contexts. Matt J. Dunn's *Dictionary of Eye Care and Vision Science* is a concise quick-reference glossary covering topics including ocular anatomy and physiology, optics, clinical techniques, pathology, low vision, orthoptics, perception, and psychophysics, as well as contemporary clinical and research terminology. Focusing on specialised terminology, this dictionary is valuable to students, clinicians, and researchers across optometry, ophthalmology, orthoptics, and vision science, as well as related fields including medical education and visual rehabilitation.

KEY FEATURES:

- Provides clear, concise definitions to immediately provide essential facts without the complexity of textbook-style material.
- Covers terminology spanning established areas and newer developments, including topics such as eye tracking.
- Structured for quick-reference use in both academic and clinical settings, supporting rapid familiarisation with technical terminology.

Dictionary of Eye Care and Vision Science

Matt J. Dunn

CRC Press
Taylor & Francis Group
Boca Raton London New York

CRC Press is an imprint of the
Taylor & Francis Group, an **informa** business

Designed cover image: Matt J. Dunn

First edition published 2027
by CRC Press
2385 NW Executive Center Drive, Suite 320, Boca Raton FL 33431

and by CRC Press
4 Park Square, Milton Park, Abingdon, Oxon, OX14 4RN

CRC Press is an imprint of Taylor & Francis Group, LLC

Library of Congress Control Number: 2026939936

ISBN: 9781041351191 (hbk)
ISBN: 9781041337065 (pbk)
ISBN: 9781003796176 (ebk)

DOI: 10.1201/9781003796176

Typeset in Minion
by Deanta Global Publishing Services, Chennai, India

PREFACE

Matt J. Dunn's *Dictionary of Eye Care and Vision Science* is a glossary of specialised terminology used in optometry, ophthalmology, and vision science, containing over 3,800 entries. It is designed as a quick-reference resource, providing clear definitions to support learning and clinical practice. This book is intended to complement more detailed texts and is suitable for students, clinicians, and vision scientists.

The focus is on advanced terminology rather than foundational vocabulary, and definitions are deliberately brief to provide the most important facts at a glance.

Topics covered include ocular anatomy and physiology, ocular pathology, optics, refraction, clinical techniques, perception, psychophysics, low vision, and orthoptics.

AUTHOR

Matt J. Dunn is Senior Lecturer in Vision Science at Cardiff University and a qualified optometrist. His research in psychophysics and neurocybernetics focuses on perceptual disorders, compensation of eye movements, and clinical applications of eye tracking technology. He is the founder of the International Society for Clinical Eye Tracking (ISCET). This book builds on his widely used digital reference resource developed to support students and clinicians.

A

A pattern
Increased **divergence** in **depression** of ≥10 **prism dioptres**. Should be classified as A(**eso**) or A(**exo**).

a-wave
Negative peak in **electroretinography** primarily caused by photoreceptors. Larger and slower in dark-adapted individuals.

a.c.
Acronym of ante cibum (before meals).

AAION
*Acronym of **arteritic anterior ischaemic optic neuropathy**.*

Abbe value
*Synonym of **constringence**.*

abducens nerve
Innervates the ipsilateral **lateral rectus**. *Synonym is **sixth cranial nerve**.*

abduct
*Verb form of **abduction**.*

abduction
Eye movement in a temporal direction. *Verb form is **abduct**.*

aberration
Any imperfection in the image formed by an optical system. There are two major types: monochromatic aberration and **chromatic aberration**.

abnormal head posture
A head posture that is adopted to compensate for problems such as **extraocular muscle** palsies (to bring the diplopic images together or separate them as much as possible); **nystagmus** (to put the eyes in the **null position**); or neck and postural problems. *Acronym is **AHP**. Synonyms are **compensatory head posture** and **ocular torticollis**.*

abnormal retinal correspondence
*Synonym of **anomalous retinal correspondence**.*

abrasion
Damage to the skin, no deeper than the epidermis.

absolute scotoma
A **scotoma** in which there is no sensitivity to any brightness whatsoever.

absolute subjective visual direction
Visual direction that is calculated taking into account both head and eye position. *Synonym is **egocentric subjective visual direction**.*

absolute threshold
In **psychophysics**, the minimum stimulus intensity that can be perceived. Low threshold = high sensitivity.

AC
*Acronym of **anterior chamber**.*

AC/A
*Acronym of **accommodative convergence:accommodation ratio**.*

acanthamoeba
A non-parasitic protozoan. Swimming in contact lenses, rinsing contact lenses with tap water, and trauma all increase the risk of infection.

Acc
*Abbreviation of **accommodation**.*

accessory optic nuclei
Regions of the **optic tract** involved in **optic flow**. Large **receptive fields** detect **retinal slip**, inducing **optokinetic nystagmus**. *Synonym is **accessory optic system**.*

accessory optic system
*Synonym of **accessory optic nuclei**.*

Accomm
*Abbreviation of **accommodation**.*

accommodate
*Verb form of **accommodation**.*

accommodation
Contraction of the **ciliary muscle**, usually in response to a near target. *Abbreviations are **Acc** and **Accomm**. Verb form is **accommodate**.*

accommodative amplitude
*Synonym of **amplitude of accommodation**.*

accommodative convergence
The change in **convergence** elicited in response to a change in **accommodation**.

accommodative convergence:accommodation ratio

The amount of **convergence** (measured in **prism dioptres** of convergence) divided by the amount of **accommodation** (measured in **dioptres**) required to direct both eyes upon an object. Calculated using the **gradient method** or **phoria method**. *Acronym is **AC/A**.*

accommodative facility

The level of ability to use and control the available **accommodation**. Quantified using jump **convergence** testing. 10 cycles/min normal for adults; 6–7 cycles/min normal for children. *Synonym is **facility of accommodation**.*

accommodative fatigue

Tired accommodative system due to overexertion (e.g. during accommodative exercises or extensive near work).

accommodative inertia

Bilateral failure/delay in **accommodation** adapting to viewing distance. May be **Adie's pupil** if **unilateral**.

accommodative insufficiency

Having a significantly lower **amplitude of accommodation** than would be expected for a patient's age.

accommodative lag

The situation in which a patient's accommodative response to a stimulus is to focus behind the stimulus. *Synonym is **underaccommodation**.*

accommodative lead

The situation in which a patient's accommodative response to a stimulus is to focus in front of the stimulus. *Synonym is **overaccommodation**.*

accommodative paralysis

Total inability to **accommodate**.

accommodative rehabilitation

Re-training to use **accommodation** with an accommodative **intraocular lens** after years without the ability to **accommodate**.

accommodative spasm

Constant contraction of the **ciliary muscle**.

acephalgic migraine

A **migraine** in which the only symptom is the perception of a visual aura. Duration is usually the same as **classic migraine**s or **common migraine**s. This type of migraine is common in patients who have suffered with classic migraines in the past. *Synonyms are **migraine sine migraine** and **visual migraine**.*

ACG

*Acronym of **angle closure glaucoma**.*

ACh
Abbreviation of acetylcholine.

achromat
A doublet of lenses causing two wavelengths to be in focus.

achromatism
Synonym of ***achromatopsia.***

achromatopia
Synonym of ***achromatopsia.***

achromatopsia
Complete inability to perceive colour; all that is perceived is varying levels of **illumination**. *Synonyms are* ***achromatism, achromatopia, colour blindness,*** *and* ***Daltonism.***

ACIOL
Acronym of ***anterior chamber intraocular lens.***

acne rosacea
Blepharitis with inflamed nose and cheeks.

acquired nystagmus
Nystagmus that develops in response to disease or injury.

acquired primary lacrimal deficiency
Synonym of ***senile hyposecretion.***

actinic keratosis
Precancerous skin **lesion** resulting from chronic sun exposure. Rough, scaly. More common in light-skinned individuals and the elderly.

action blindsight
Form of **blindsight** in which patients are able to perform motor actions (such as **saccade**s or pointing) towards stimuli in a **visual field** defect, despite lacking conscious awareness.

activated phosphodiesterase
Converts cyclic guanosine monophosphate to 5' guanosine monophosphate.

acuity
Synonym of ***visual acuity.***

acuity reserve
The **visual acuity** of a patient as a ratio to what they can comfortably read for an extended period of time. Usually around 3:1.

A

acutance
In photography, the **contrast** at edges in an image. Can be artificially enhanced using an unsharp mask.

acute angle closure glaucoma
Pain, vomiting, and loss of vision as a result of rapidly increasing **intraocular pressure** due to closure of the **anterior chamber angle**.

acute spastic entropion
Severe **blepharospasm** causing occasional **entropion**.

acute uveitis
Uveitis that lasts less than three months.

AD
Acronym of autosomal dominant.

adaptation
The rate at which the retinas alter their sensitivity to changes in **illumination**. *Synonyms are **dark adaptation** and **light adaptation**.*

adaptive optics
Principle used to correct higher-order **aberrations** through the use of deformable mirrors which counteract waveform distortion. *Acronym is **AO**.*

add
*Synonym of **addition**.*

addition
The difference in spherical refractive correction required between an individual's distance and near prescription. *Synonyms are **add** and **reading addition**.*

additive colour production
Colour produced as a result of multiple sources of filtered white light added together.

additive Grassman's law
When equal radiation is added to both sides of metameric colour match, the match holds.

adduct
*Verb form of **adduction**.*

adduction
Eye movement in a nasal direction. *Verb form is **adduct**.*

adenoma
Cancer of glandular or duct cells.

adenovirus
Very contagious family of viruses.

adherence syndrome
*Synonym of **Johnson's adherence syndrome**.*

Adie's pupil
All **pupil** reactions are slowed (especially light), but long exposure causes overreaction. Due to peripheral nervous system **lesion**. Affected pupil is larger. Can affect just a segment of the pupil. Pupil can be dilated with **pilocarpine**. *Synonyms are **Adie's tonic pupil**, **Holmes–Adie tonic pupil**, and **tonic pupil**.*

Adie's tonic pupil
*Synonym of **Adie's pupil**.*

adjustable sutures
A type of suture sometimes used in **strabismus** surgery so that the ocular angle can be altered after the surgery is complete.

adnexa
The appendages of an organ. In reference to the eyes, this generally describes the **extraocular muscles**, **eyelids**, and **lacrimal glands**.

ADOA
*Acronym of **autosomal dominant optic atrophy**.*

ADR
Acronym of adverse drug reaction.

adult Best's disease
*Synonym of **adult vitelliform disease**.*

adult vitelliform disease
Best vitelliform macular dystrophy when it presents in the 4th–5th decades of life (Best's presents in 1st decade). *Synonym is **adult Best's disease**.*

advanced surface ablation
*Synonym of **photorefractive keratectomy**.*

adventitious blindness
Any blindness which is acquired during life (i.e. not **congenital**).

aesthesiometer
Device used to measure **corneal touch threshold**.

aesthetic colour judging
Knowing which colours work well together.

A

afferent nerve
A nerve that carries a signal towards the central nervous system. *Opposite of **efferent nerve**.*

afferent pupillary defect
*Synonym of **relative afferent pupillary defect**.*

afibrinogenemia
Complete lack of **fibrinogen**, therefore no clotting of blood.

aflibercept
An anti-**VEGF** treatment delivered **intravitreal**ly for **wet age-related macular degeneration**, **retinal vein occlusion**, and diabetic **macula**r oedema.

after-nystagmus
*Synonym of **optokinetic after-nystagmus**.*

afterimage
The persistence of perception of an image on the retina after the original stimulus is removed.

afterimage test
Flashes of light are presented to each eye separately: one horizontal, one vertical. The subjective **afterimage** can be used to indicate the state of binocularity.

against-the-rule astigmatism
Astigmatism in which the negative **axis** is within 15° either side of vertical (90°); the steepest meridian is horizontal. *Acronym is **atr**.*

AGE
Acronym of advanced glycation endproduct.

age-related macular degeneration
Age-related damage to the **macula**. There are two types: **dry age-related macular degeneration** and **wet age-related macular degeneration**. The types are classified by the nature of the damage. *Acronyms are **AMD** and **ARMD**. Synonyms are **macular degeneration** and **senile macular degeneration**.*

age-related maculopathy
Few **soft drusen** with **retinal pigment epithelium** abnormalities (hyper/hypopigmentation). Not severe enough to be classified as **age-related macular degeneration**. *Acronym is **ARM**.*

agenesis
Failure of an organ to develop.

aggregate field
*Synonym of **location column**.*

agnosia
*Synonym of **visual agnosia**.*

agnosopsia
The ability to make better-than-chance judgements about stimuli, without conscious awareness. A type of **blindsight**. *Opposite of* ***gnosanopsia***.

agraphia
Synonym of ***dysgraphia***.

AHP
Acronym of ***abnormal head posture***.

AI
Acronym of ***artificial intelligence***.

AIDS
Acronym of acquired immunodeficiency syndrome.

AIDS retinopathy
Cotton wool spots, haemorrhages, **microaneurysms**. Does not correlate with the level of immunodeficiency. *Synonyms are* ***HIV retinal microangiopathy*** *and* ***HIV retinopathy***.

AIK
Acronym of asymptomatic ***sterile infiltrative keratitis***.

AION
Acronym of ***anterior ischaemic optic neuropathy***.

Airy disc
The patch of light that actually reaches the retina. Wider in the periphery due to lens **aberrations**.

AK
Acronym of ***astigmatic keratotomy***.

Akahoshi chopper
Device that cleaves a **cataract** into two, allowing for more speedy surgical removal.

AKC
Acronym of ***atopic keratoconjunctivitis***.

akinetopsia
Inability to perceive movement of any kind, due to damage to **hMT+**. *Synonyms are* ***cerebral akinetopsia*** *and* ***motion blindness***.

Åland Island disease
Rare X-linked condition with **fundus** hypopigmentation and foveal dysplasia. Causes poor visual acuity, **fusion maldevelopment nystagmus syndrome**, progressive myopia, **protan** defects, and **nyctalopia**. *Synonym is* ***Forsius–Eriksson syndrome***.

A

albinism
Either **ocular albinism** or **oculocutaneous albinism**; in both cases, the eyes are hypopigmented.

albino
An individual affected by **albinism**.

Alexander's law
When an individual with **vestibular nystagmus** looks in the direction of the **nystagmus** quick phase, **nystagmus intensity** increases. Also applies in **fusion maldevelopment nystagmus syndrome**.

alexia without agraphia
*Synonym of **pure alexia**.*

aliasing
Describes the situation in which, due to undersampling, a stimulus can be detected but whose form is unresolvable.

Alice in Wonderland syndrome
Perceptual disturbance causing **metamorphopsia**, **dysmetropsia**, **chromatopsia**, and altered self-body image (distortion of perceived body part size/shape). Believed to be more frequent in young children; can be a form of **migraine aura**, a side-effect of hallucinogenic drug intoxication, an early sign of Epstein–Barr virus infection, or brain tumour. Symptoms occur more frequently around the onset of sleep. Although some sufferers simply 'grow out of' the condition, referral is required to rule out life-threatening causes. *Synonym is **Todd's syndrome**.*

aligning prism
*Synonym of **associated phoria**.*

all-trans-retinal
Chromophore present in metarhodopsin II.

all-trans-retinol
Converted from **all-trans-retinal**. Migrates to the **retinal pigment epithelium** to become 11-cis-retinal.

allergic conjunctivitis
Inflammation of the **conjunctiva** due to allergy. There are three types: **atopic keratoconjunctivitis**, **allergic rhinoconjunctivitis**, and **vernal keratoconjunctivitis**. *Synonym is **atopic conjunctivitis**.*

allergic rhinoconjunctivitis
A form of **allergic conjunctivitis**. Transient swelling and **chemosis**. Itching. Nasal symptoms.

allocentric unilateral neglect
Unilateral neglect of spatial relationships between objects.

alpha crystallins
Molecular chaperone for beta and gamma crystallins in the lens.

Alport syndrome
A basement membrane disorder that causes **cataract**, **posterior polymorphous dystrophy**, **anterior lenticonus**, and deafness.

Alström syndrome
Rare genetic disorder, sometimes confused with **Bardet–Biedl syndrome.** Causes **nystagmus** and **photophobia**.

ALT
Acronym of ***argon laser trabeculoplasty.***

alternating contact lens
Synonym of ***translating contact lens.***

alternating hyperphoria
Synonym of ***dissociated vertical deviation.***

alternating vision contact lens
Synonym of ***translating contact lens.***

altitudinal visual field defect
A **visual field** defect predominantly above or below the **raphé**.

amacrine cell
Cell type present in the **inner plexiform layer**, **inner nuclear layer**, and, to a small extent, the **ganglion cell layer**, which connect **bipolar cells** and **ganglion cells**.

amaurosis
Vision loss without a **lesion**.

amaurosis fugax
A transient **monocular** visual loss.

amaurotic pupil
Describes an eye with an absolute afferent **pupil** defect.

ambiguous picture
An image which may be interpreted in multiple ways; only one perception can occur at a time.

amblyope
An individual affected by **amblyopia**.

A

amblyopia
Reduced sensitivity of an eye due to reduced input during the **plastic period**. *Adjective form is **amblyopic**. Synonym is **lazy eye**.*

amblyopia ex anopsia
Refers to **strabismic amblyopia** or **stimulus deprivation amblyopia**.

amblyopic
*Adjective form of **amblyopia**.*

amblyoscope
A device used to train an **amblyopic** eye, encouraging its use in binocular vision.

AMD
*Acronym of **age-related macular degeneration**.*

Ames room
A visual illusion in which a seemingly normal room has sloping walls so that objects placed at one end seem smaller, rather than further away.

amethocaine
*Synonym of **tetracaine**.*

ametropia
Any refractive error.

amide-linked anaesthetic
Degraded slower than **ester-linked anaesthetic**, as must be metabolised by the liver. Lasts ~30–60 mins. **Lidocaine** is an example.

amiodarone keratopathy
*Synonym of **corneal verticillata**.*

amplitude of accommodation
The highest amount of **accommodation** that an eye can produce, recorded in **dioptres**. Typically measured using the **push up method**, **push down method**, or **dynamic retinoscopy**. Can also be measured by determining the amount of **minus lens** that can be tolerated without blur in addition to the distance prescription. *Synonym is **accommodative amplitude**.*

ampulla
Structure in each **semicircular canal** that excites the **vestibular nerve** when fluid passes the **kinocilia** in one direction. *Plural is **ampullae**. Synonym is **osseous ampulla**.*

ampullae
*Plural of **ampulla**.*

Amsler grid
A grid of 400 squares with a central **fixation** spot, used to detect **metamorphopsia** or positive **scotomata**. There are many designs available, including black-on-white, white-on-black, red-on-black, and those with a diagonal line designed to help localise the fixation spot in the presence of a central **scotoma**.

anaemia
Reduced haemoglobin count/low blood oxygen. A complication of **leukaemia**.

anaglyph
A 3D image composed of two colours, usually red and blue.

anastomosis
Connection between blood vessels.

anatomical bridge
*Synonym of **comfort bridge**.*

Anderson–Kestenbaum surgery
*Synonym of **Kestenbaum surgery**.*

aneuploidy
A change in the number of chromosomes. Common in cancerous cells.

aneurysm
A localised bulge in a blood vessel. Can burst at any time.

angiogenesis
Growth of blood vessels from pre-existing vessels.

angioid streaks
Streaks (damaged **Bruch's membrane**) from the **optic nerve head** to midperipheral **fundus** with **drusen**. Due to disrupted **choriocapillaris**.

angioscotoma
The image of the retinal blood vessels that is normally suppressed by the brain. It can often be seen when a high-intensity focused light is shone on the retina (for example during **ophthalmoscopy**). *Synonym is **Purkinje tree**.*

angle alpha
The angle between the optical and visual axes of the eye. Usually ~5° positive. A larger positive angle gives the appearance of nasally displaced **corneal reflexes**, causing pseudoexotropia. Similar, but not identical, to **angle kappa**.

angle closure glaucoma
*Synonym of **closed angle glaucoma**.*

A

angle kappa
The angle between the pupillary and visual axes of the eye. A large positive angle gives the appearance of nasally displaced **corneal reflex**es, causing pseudoexotropia. Similar, but not identical, to **angle alpha**. *Synonym is **kappa angle**.*

angle of incidence
The angle between a ray incident on a surface and the **normal**.

angle of reflection
The angle between a ray reflected from a surface and the **normal**.

angular dispersion
The angle formed by red and blue emergent light dispersed through a prism.

angular magnification
*Synonym of **telescopic magnification**.*

anhidrosis
Lack of sweating.

aniridia
Absence of the iris.

aniseikonia
A difference between each eye in the image sizes at the retinas, usually caused by **anisometropia**. If significantly different, can cause difficulties in maintaining **sensory fusion**.

anisocoria
Unequal **pupil** sizes.

anisometropia
A difference in refractive error between the two eyes.

anisometropic amblyopia
Stimulus deprivation amblyopia as a result of uncorrected **anisometropia**. **Amblyopia** is typically in the most hyperopic eye.

anisophoria
A **phoria** that is **incomitant**.

ankyloblepharon
Eyelids joined together, for example by scarring.

ankylosing spondylitis
Condition causing gradual fusion of the spine. *Synonyms are **Marie–Strümpell disease** and **rheumatoid spondylitis**.*

annular
Having the form of a ring.

annular tendon
Synonym of ***annulus of Zinn.***

annulus of Zinn
Tendinous ring around the **optic nerve**; source of the rectus **extraocular muscles** and **superior oblique**. Surrounded by the **circle of Zinn–Haller**. *Synonyms are* ***annular tendon*** *and* ***common tendinous ring.***

anomaloscope
Device used to measure colour vision.

anomalous retinal correspondence
Condition in which the **fovea** of one eye is associated with an area other than the fovea of the other eye. Develops as an **adaptation** in small-angle **strabismus** to prevent **diplopia** and **confusion**. Classified into **harmonious anomalous retinal correspondence, unharmonious anomalous retinal correspondence**, and **paradoxical anomalous retinal correspondence.** *Acronym is* ***ARC****. Synonym is* ***abnormal retinal correspondence.***

anomalous trichromatism
Condition in which all three photoreceptor types are present, but one does not work well.

anophthalmia
Failure of one or both eyes to develop during embryological development. *Synonym is* ***anophthalmos.***

anophthalmos
Synonym of ***anophthalmia.***

anopsia
A complete lack of vision (such as in a typical **visual field** defect).

anosognosia
Describes the situation in which a patient is unaware of their own disability. **Anton syndrome** is an example.

anoxia
Complete lack of oxygen.

ANS
Acronym of autonomic nervous system.

anterior basement membrane dystrophy
Synonym of ***Cogan's microcystic dystrophy.***

A

anterior blepharitis
Blepharitis: specifically, **inflammation** of **lash** follicles, **Moll glands**, or **Zeis glands**.

anterior chamber
The part of the eye delineated by the front of the lens and the back of the **cornea**. *Acronym is AC.*

anterior chamber angle
The angle formed by the junction of the iris and the **cornea**. *Synonym is **iridocorneal angle**.*

anterior chamber intraocular lens
An **intraocular lens** that is placed in the **anterior chamber** (in rare cases where not possible in the old lens **capsule**). *Acronym is **ACIOL**.*

anterior choroidal artery
Artery that branches from the middle cerebral artery. Supplies the **optic chiasm, optic tract, lateral geniculate nucleus**, and **optic radiations**.

anterior ischaemic optic neuropathy
Occurs in individuals between 45 and 85 years of age. Causes an altitudinal **visual field** defect. There are two types: **arteritic anterior ischaemic optic neuropathy** and **non-arteritic anterior ischaemic optic neuropathy**. *Acronyms are **AION** and **ION**.*

anterior lenticonus
A bulge in the anterior crystalline lens.

anterior synechia
Adhesion of the iris to the **cornea**.

anterior uvea
The anterior **ciliary body** and iris.

anterior uveitis
Inflammation of the **anterior uvea**.

antimetropia
The case in which one eye is myopic and the other hyperopic.

antisaccade
The situation in which a contraversive **saccade** is made away from the direction of a visual target (as opposed to a **prosaccade** towards it). Used as a clinical test of voluntary motor control.

Anton syndrome
Form of **anosognosia** characterised by denial of blindness following bilateral **V1** damage, despite being totally cortically blind. *Synonym is **Anton–Babinski syndrome**.*

Anton–Babinski syndrome
*Synonym of **Anton syndrome**.*

AO
*Acronym of **adaptive optics**.*

AOS
*Acronym of **accessory optic system**.*

APD
*Acronym of **afferent pupillary defect**.*

aperiodic alternating nystagmus
Periodic alternating nystagmus with a varying period duration.

aperture
The size of a hole through which light is permitted.

aphakia
Condition in which an eye does not have a lens, neither crystalline or pseudophakic.

aphakic intraocular lens
An **intraocular lens** when it is the only lens in a patient's eye.

aphantasia
Inability to experience **visual imagery**.

apical angle
The angle made by the apex of a prism.

aplasia
Failure of part of an organ to develop.

apochromat
At least two lenses which together cause three wavelengths of light to be in focus.

apostilb
A unit of brightness. 1 apostilb = $1/\pi$ cd/m^2. Unit = asb.

apparent motion
Perceived motion when there is no real movement of a stimulus. There are two types: **beta motion** and **phi motion**.

apperceptive prosopagnosia
Prosopagnosia in which the patient is completely unable to distinguish features such as gender and emotion from faces. Compare with **associative prosopagnosia**.

apperceptive visual agnosia
Visual agnosia due to the inability to perceive a structured whole. Compare with **associative visual agnosia**.

applanate
*Verb form of **applanation**.*

applanation
Flattening. *Verb form is **applanate**.*

applanation tonometer
Instrument used in **applanation tonometry**.

applanation tonometry
Tonometry that uses the principle of measuring the force required to **applanate** the **cornea** in order to judge **intraocular pressure**. The **Perkins tonometer** and **Goldmann tonometer** are common examples of this type of **tonometer**.

Aq
*Abbreviation of **aqueous humour**.*

aqueous humour
The fluid present in the **anterior chamber** of the eye. *Abbreviation is **Aq**.*

aqueous layer
The middle layer of the tear film containing water, inorganic salts, glucose, urea, proteins, and **glycoproteins**. *Synonym is **lacrimal layer**.*

AR
*Acronym of anti-reflection/**augmented reality**/autosomal recessive.*

arachnoid
The central **meninx**. Resembles a spider's web. *Synonym is **arachnoid mater**.*

arachnoid mater
*Synonym of **arachnoid**.*

ARC
*Acronym of **anomalous retinal correspondence**.*

arc-eye
*Synonym of **photokeratitis**.*

arcuate fibres
In the retina, the fibres that come from beyond the **fovea**.

arcuate scotoma
A **scotoma** that follows the path of the retinal nerve fibres from the **optic nerve head** into the nasal **visual field**. *Synonyms are **Bjerrum scotoma** and **Seidel scotoma**.*

arcus
*Synonym of **arcus senilis**.*

arcus juvenilis
Arcus senilis when it occurs in a younger patient; indicative of **hypercholesterolaemia**. Also known as 'juvenile arcus'.

arcus lipoides
*Synonym of **arcus senilis**.*

arcus senilis
A milky coloured arc at the **limbus** due to **lipid** deposition frequently seen after age 50. May be a sign of **hypercholesterolaemia**. *Synonyms are **arcus**, **arcus lipoides**, **corneal arcus**, **gerontoxon**, and **senile arcus**.*

Arden index
The ratio of the light peak to the dark peak in **electro-oculography**, expressed as a percentage. <180% suggests **retinal pigment epithelium** disease. *Synonym is **Arden ratio**.*

Arden ratio
*Synonym of **Arden index**.*

ARE
*Acronym of **contact lens induced acute red eye**.*

argon laser trabeculoplasty
Tiny burns made all over the **trabecular meshwork** in an attempt to reduce **intraocular pressure**. *Acronym is **ALT**.*

Argyll Robertson pupil
Anisocoria and **light-near dissociation**. Caused by brain damage/syphilis. *Synonym is **prostitute's pupil**.*

ARM
*Acronym of **age-related maculopathy**.*

ARMD
*Acronym of **age-related macular degeneration**.*

Arnold–Chiari malformation
A malformation of the brain. Can cause **nystagmus**, **strabismus**, and **dysmetric saccades**, as well as difficulties with **smooth pursuit** and **vestibulo-ocular reflex**. *Synonym is **Chiari malformation**.*

A

arteriolosclerosis
Loss of elasticity (hardening) of arterioles. Often due to **hypertension**.

arteriosclerosis
Loss of elasticity (hardening) of medium or large arteries.

arteritic anterior ischaemic optic neuropathy
Pallor and **oedema** of the **optic disc**, few splinter haemorrhages, hyperfluorescent **fundus fluorescein angiography**. Caused by **giant cell arteritis**. Requires speedy referral. Also known as 'arteritic anterior ischaemic optic neuropathy'. *Acronym is* ***AAION***.

arthralgia
Pain in the joints.

artificial intelligence
The ability for a computer system to undertake tasks that would normally require human intelligence, such as interpreting medical images and making diagnostic decisions. *Acronym is* ***AI***.

artificial neural network
Synonym of ***neural network***.

ASA
Acronym of ***advanced surface ablation***.

ASC
Acronym of anterior subcapsular lens opacity.

ASD
Acronym of autistic spectrum disorder.

aseptic keratitis
Synonym of ***sterile infiltrative keratitis***.

assistive technology
Any technology that supports people with a disability. Includes **low vision aids**. *Acronym is* *AT*.

associated phoria
The amount of prism correction required to neutralise a **fixation disparity**. This may be greater than the size of the fixation disparity, but never greater than the total **heterophoria**. *Synonym is* ***aligning prism***.

associative prosopagnosia
Prosopagnosia in which the patient is able to distinguish features such as gender and emotion in faces, but is unable to recognise who they are. Compare with **apperceptive prosopagnosia**.

associative visual agnosia
Visual agnosia due to the inability to associate visual objects with a semantic meaning from memory. Compare with **apperceptive visual agnosia**.

astatikopsia
Synonym of ***statokinetic dissociation***.

astereopsis
Complete lack of **stereopsis**. May occur as a result of damage to the posterior parietal lobe.

asteroid hyalosis
Soapy looking debris (calcium particles) in the **vitreous humour.**

asthenopia
Generalised, non-specific eye strain. This can include soreness, blurred vision, headaches, redness of the eyes, general tiredness, **diplopia**, etc. A symptom of excessive concentrated work.

astigmatic amblyopia
Synonym of ***meridional amblyopia***.

astigmatic keratotomy
Refractive surgery in which an incision is made on the steep **axis** of the **cornea,** peripheral to the **pupil** zone, to correct up to ~3.00 DC of corneal **astigmatism**. *Acronym is AK.*

astigmatism
A refractive error which requires a cylindrical correction.

astringent
Describes a chemical that causes constriction of blood vessels.

astronomical telescope
Synonym of ***Keplerian telescope***.

AT
Acronym of ***assistive technology***.

Athens protocol
Keratoconus treatment protocol involving **photorefractive keratectomy** and **collagen cross-linking** being performed on the same day.

atheroma
A **plaque** (accumulation of debris) inside an artery.

atherosclerosis
Arteriosclerosis when it is due to a **plaque** (the most common type of arteriosclerosis).

atopic conjunctivitis
*Synonym of **allergic conjunctivitis**.*

atopic dermatitis
A type of eczema. Associated with **keratoconus**.

atopic keratoconjunctivitis
A form of **allergic conjunctivitis**. Loss of features on the **tarsal conjunctiva**. **Symblepharon**. Punctate staining. Peripheral **neovascularisation**. *Acronym is **AKC**.*

atopy
A predisposition to an allergic reaction.

atoric
Describes an aspheric form of a toric surface.

atr
*Acronym of **against-the-rule astigmatism**.*

atrophic age-related macular degeneration
*Synonym of **dry age-related macular degeneration**.*

atrophic round hole
A common peripheral retinal degeneration. In very rare cases can lead to a **retinal detachment**.

atropine
An antimuscarinic **cycloplegic**.

attentional blindsight
*Synonym of **Riddoch phenomenon**.*

Aubert–Fleischl phenomenon
The perceived movement of a target when not tracking it is 70% of the actual movement.

augmented reality
Form of **extended reality** in which the user wears a **head-mounted display** which allows a partial view of the real world. May be used as a **low vision aid**. *Synonym is **mixed reality**.*

autosomal dominant optic atrophy
*Synonym of **dominant optic atrophy**.*

autosome
A chromosome that is neither X nor Y.

avascular
Lacking a blood supply.

Avellino dystrophy
Synonym of ***granular dystrophy type III****.*

avulsion
An injury leading to an exposed flap of skin.

Axenfeld loops
A fairly common abnormality of the **sclera,** seen as a raised pigmented area. Due to the long ciliary nerve looping in an anomalous fashion. Differentiate from tumour. *Synonym is* ***loops of Axenfeld****.*

axial ametropia
Ametropia caused by the length of the eye. Can cause **optical aniseikonia.**

axial plane
Synonym of ***transverse plane****.*

axis
The angle in degrees of one of two major meridians a prescribed cylindrical power acts in.

AZOOR
Acronym of acute zonal occult outer retinopathy.

B

b-wave
Positive peak in **electroretinography** due to **Müller cells** and ON-**bipolar cell**s. Larger and slower in dark-adapted individuals.

b.i.d.
Acronym of bis in die (twice daily).

back optic zone diameter
The total diameter of the back optic zone of a contact lens. In order to maintain a stable RGP lens fit, flatten the **back optic zone radius** by 0.05 mm for every 0.50 mm increase in back optic zone diameter. *Acronym is **BOZD**.*

back optic zone radius
*Synonym of **base curve**.*

back vertex distance
The distance between the front of the **cornea** and the back of a spectacle lens. *Acronym is **BVD**. Synonym is **vertex distance**.*

back vertex power
The effective power of a lens at the back surface of a lens. *Acronym is **BVP**. Synonym is **vertex power**.*

background diabetic retinopathy
Microaneurysms, haemorrhages, **hard exudates**, retinal oedema. *Acronym is **BDR**.*

bacterial conjunctivitis
Conjunctivitis with a mucopurulent discharge. Usually treated with broad spectrum antibiotics.

bactericidal
Describes antibiotics that kill bacteria.

bacteriostatic
Describes antibiotics that slow the growth or reproduction of bacteria.

bagging
The unscrupulous practice of putting a lens in a plastic bag to make it fit into a frame (when glazed too small). The excess bag is then cut away.

Bagolini filter bar
*Synonym of **Sbisa bar**.*

Bagolini glasses
Lenses used to assess **simultaneous perception** and whether **anomalous retinal correspondence** is present. Like a very fine **Maddox rod**, the lenses don't dissociate the eyes but cause light points to be seen as streaks.

Bailey–Lovie chart
A **logMAR** chart calibrated for use at 6 metres. Lower **contrast** versions are available.

Bálint–Holmes syndrome
*Synonym of **Bálint's syndrome**.*

Bálint's syndrome
Bilateral damage to parietal cortex, causing **saccade initiation failure, simultanagnosia**, and **optic ataxia**. Patients exhibit **spatial disorientation**. *Synonym is **Bálint–Holmes syndrome**.*

band keratopathy
Calcium deposits on the **cornea**.

bandage contact lens
A contact lens that is worn to help the **cornea** heal.

bandwidth (spatial frequency)
The ratio of spatial frequencies at which **contrast sensitivity** is halved.

Bangerter foil
A thin layer of vinyl that can be attached to the front of a spectacle lens to reduce form perception. Used in **amblyopia** therapy.

bar magnifier
A type of **bright field magnifier** that magnifies in one direction only. Useful for reading whole lines of text.

Bardet–Biedl syndrome
A condition characterised by obesity and mental retardation that is often associated with **retinitis pigmentosa**.

Barrer units
*Synonym of **Fatt units**.*

Barrett retinoscopy
Method of performing **retinoscopy** for **monocular** practitioners (as being on **axis** will be more difficult for one of the eyes). The patient fixates on the **retinoscope** light, and the reflex is neutralised. Then, the patient focuses in the distance and the procedure is repeated. This gives the **accommodation**, which is added to the result from the first measure.

basal cell carcinoma
Common skin cancer. Usually on the face, rarely malignant. Two main types frequently occur in ophthalmology: noduloulcerative (**rodent ulcer**) and sclerosing. *Acronym is **BCC**.*

B

basal cell papilloma
Very common skin lesion found in middle-aged to elderly patients. Dark, well-circumscribed, painless, usually elevated, not malignant.

basal laminar drusen
Synonym of ***cuticular drusen***.

basal tears
The natural, unstimulated tears that keep the **cornea** nourished. Secreted at a rate of approximately 1 μl/minute and 1.5 ml/day. Turnover is roughly 16%/minute.

base curve
1. In an ophthalmic lens, the difference between the **cross curve** and base curve = lens cylinder power.
2. When referring to contact lenses, the radius of curvature of the back surface of the lens. To maintain the fit of a **rigid gas permeable** contact lens, every 0.05 mm base curve increase should be accompanied by adding +0.25 D to the **back vertex power**. *Acronym is BC. Synonym is* ***back optic zone radius***.

Basedow–Graves disease
Synonym of ***Graves' disease***.

Bates method
An outdated set of alternative therapies intended to improve visual function, including ocular exercises to improve refractive error, visualisation techniques, and relaxation by covering the eyes with the hands. Many of the techniques have been proven to be ineffective, and some, such as focusing the sun directly onto the eye with a lens, are considered dangerous.

Bausch and Lomb keratometer
A type of **one position keratometer**.

BC
Acronym of ***base curve***.

BCC
Acronym of ***basal cell carcinoma***.

BD
Acronym of base down.

BDR
Acronym of ***background diabetic retinopathy***.

BE
Acronym of both eyes.

bear track pigmentation
Multiple **congenital choroidal hypertrophy** lesions on the **fundus**. Looks like paw prints.

behavioural inattention test
A set of tests designed to screen for **unilateral neglect**. *Synonym is* ***Rivermead behavioural inattention test***.

Bell's palsy
Idiopathic partial **palsy** of **facial nerve,** resulting in lack of control of face on affected side. Poor **eyelid** closure.

Bell's phenomenon
The phenomenon present in some individuals that causes an outward and upward rolling of the eyes when closing or attempting to close the eyes. *Synonym is* ***palpebral oculogyric reflex***.

benary cross
An equal-luminance visual illusion which defies explanation by **contrast** changes.

benign familial fleck retina
Yellow to white flecks throughout **fundus** (except at **fovea**). Rare, asymptomatic.

benign intracranial hypertension
Synonym of ***idiopathic intracranial hypertension***.

benign paroxysmal positional vertigo
Inner ear disorder causing **positional nystagmus**.

benign tumour
A tumour that is slow spreading, not necessarily dangerous unless in an unfortunate place.

benoxinate
Synonym of ***oxybuprocaine***.

Benson's syndrome
Synonym of ***posterior cortical atrophy***.

Berger's postlenticular space
The space between the posterior lens and the **hyaloid vessel**. *Synonym is* ***retrolental space of Erggelet***.

Bergmeister's papilla
A remnant of the **hyaloid vessel** at the **optic nerve head**.

Bernard–Horner syndrome
Synonym of ***Horner's syndrome***.

best form lens
A lens designed to control **oblique astigmatism**.

Best vitelliform macular dystrophy
An inherited **retinal pigment epithelium** and macular disease. Typically occurs in individuals <10 years of age. Signs are an 'egg-yolk' **macula**, pseudo**hypopyon**, and a reduced light peak as measured with **electro-oculography**. *Synonym is **Best's disease**.*

Best's disease
*Synonym of **Best vitelliform macular dystrophy**.*

beta motion
Apparent motion of a stimulus that is flashed in two retinal locations in quick succession.

Beyne lantern
A **lantern test** that is used in France.

BHTT
*Acronym of **Bielschowsky head tilt test**.*

BI
Acronym of base in.

bi-medial recessions
Weakening operation performed on the medial recti by reinserting them more posteriorly – cures **convergence esotropia**, near **esotropia**, etc.

Biederman's recognition by components theory
Theory of object recognition that states that all 3D shapes are broken into **geons**. This theory allows for **viewpoint invariance**.

Bielschowsky head tilt test
Step 3 of the **Parks' three-step test**, commonly used to identify **palsy** of the **trochlear nerve**. The head is tilted to both sides to determine which side maximises vertical **diplopia**. Either the **SO** or **SR** of the eye on this side, or the **IO** or **IR** on the other side, is affected. For example, a trochlear nerve palsy will increase diplopia when tilting to the affected side. *Acronym is BHTT. Synonym is **head tilt test**.*

bifurcation
Splitting into two.

bilateral
On both sides.

binocular
Both eyes.

binocular cell
In the **primary visual cortex**, any cell that is not completely **monocular** (most of them) – grades 2–6, but not 1 and 7.

BIO
Acronym of binocular indirect ***ophthalmoscopy***.

bioavailability
The rate and extent of drug absorption.

biological motion
The ability to understand natural movement of organisms, especially that of humans, with very little information (such as when a silhouette is obscured). This ability is believed to develop around four months of age.

biopolymer contact lens
A contact lens made of collagen – mostly used as **bandage contact lens**es.

biopsy
Removal of tissue for examination.

bioptics
The combination of different types of refractive surgery to achieve an outcome.

biotransformation
The rate and extent of drug metabolism or degradation.

biphasic square-wave intrusion
A type of **square-wave intrusion** seen in normal patients. After fixating for a short time, a horizontal **saccade** moves the eyes off **fixation**, followed by a short pause, followed by a **hypermetric saccade** back towards the target, followed by another short pause, and finally a corrective saccade back to the target.

bipolar cell
Cell in the retina, present in the **inner plexiform layer**, **inner nuclear layer**, and **outer plexiform layer**. They synapse with photoreceptors, **ganglion cell**s, and **amacrine cell**s.

biprism bifocal
A bifocal in which there is prism incorporated into the segment as well as **slab on** or **slab off**.

biprism test
Base in and base out prisms are alternated in front of one eye during binocular fixation as an objective assessment of **motor fusion**.

birefringence
Describes the property of a material whose **refractive index** depends on the polarisation and direction of travel of light.

bitemporal hemianopia
Heteronymous hemianopia affecting the temporal side of each **visual field**. Indicative of a **lesion** at the **optic chiasm**.

Bitot's spots
Spots on the **conjunctiva**; a sign of vitamin A deficiency.

Bjerrum scotoma
Synonym of ***arcuate scotoma***.

Bjerrum screen
Synonym of ***tangent screen***.

black body
A theoretical perfect radiator of electromagnetic energy which absorbs and emits all wavelengths equally.

black body curve
Synonym of ***Planckian locus***.

black sunbursts
Hyperplasia patches of the **retinal pigment epithelium**, seen in **sickle cell retinopathy**.

blastoma
Tumour caused by abnormal precursor cells.

blebs
Swelling of the **corneal endothelium**. Appear as dark spots due to the optics with a slit lamp.

blended lenticular lens
A **lenticular lens** that has a gradual change between the refractive and carrier lenses; similar in appearance to **polynomial aspheric** lenses, but there is an area of poor optics.

blephara
Plural of ***eyelid***.

blepharitis
Group of disorders causing **inflammation** of the **eyelid** margins, **collarettes**, and dilated vessels.

blepharon
Synonym of ***eyelid***.

blepharophimosis
Congenital disorder causing **ptosis**, **telecanthus**, **epicanthus inversus**, and lower lid **ectropion**.

blepharospasm
Involuntary contraction of the muscles around the **eyelids**.

blindsight
Residual visual abilities in a 'blind' region of the visual field, usually following brain damage. There are three types: **action blindsight, attentional blindsight**, and **agnosopsia**.

blob
Areas of the **visual cortex** that stain with **cytochrome oxidase**. Indicates colour specific **parvo cells**. Located in the centre of a **hypercolumn**.

Bloch's law
Psychophysical law that states that the threshold luminance of a stimulus multiplied by the length of time the stimulus is presented for is constant, if the time is less than the **critical duration**. *Synonym is **Bunsen–Roscoe–Bloch law**.*

blot haemorrhage
A haemorrhage between the **inner nuclear layer** and the **nerve fibre layer**.

blowout fracture
Injury caused by blunt trauma in which the **orbit**al contents become squashed, causing an increase in **intraocular pressure**, often with a fractured orbital floor. If the **optic nerve head** is squashed, **visual field** loss occurs.

blue arcs phenomenon
*Synonym of **Purkinje blue arcs**.*

blue dot cataract
Congenital punctate blue **cataract**s which rarely affect vision.

blue field entoptic phenomenon
Leukocytes do not absorb as much blue light as erythrocytes. Thus, their location can be seen as an **entoptic phenomenon** of bright spots when viewed against a blue background as they pass through the **perifoveal** blood vessels. *Synonym is **Scheerer's phenomenon**.*

blue sclerans
A **congenital** thinning of the **sclera**, causing a bluish appearance to the sclera.

blur point
The minimum amount of prism that must be introduced such that vision becomes blurred due to **accommodation**.

BNX
*Acronym of **benoxinate**.*

BO
Acronym of base out.

B

Bock candy test
A gross test of near **visual acuity** in which an infant is offered some 'hundreds & thousands' cake decoration sweets to eat. Successfully reaching for and eating the sweets constitutes a pass.

bone spicule pigmentation
Retinal pigment clumping. A sign of **retinitis pigmentosa** or **retinitis punctata albescens.**

border tissue
Synonym of ***marginal tissue.***

Borrelia
Genus of bacteria that causes **Lyme's disease.** Transmitted by ticks.

botox
Synonym of ***botulinum toxin (type A).***

bottom-up processing
Model(s) of visual processing that assume the visual scene is built from smaller parts.

botulinum toxin (type A)
A product of the 'Clostridium botulinum' bacteria. Inhibits the release of acetylcholine, thereby downregulating the parasympathetic nervous system. Used as a medication, injected into muscles to temporarily reduce their action. For example, for an **exotropia**, it is injected into the lateral recti. *Synonym is* ***botox.***

Bouma's law
Within any given direction from the **fovea**, the **crowding effect** is proportional to the eccentricity at which the target stimulus is presented.

bowl lenticular
A negative **lenticular lens.**

Bowman's layer
Synonym of ***Bowman's membrane.***

Bowman's membrane
Thin **corneal** layer, between the epithelium and stroma. Smooth, made of collagen only. *Synonym is* ***Bowman's layer.***

box-carring
Synonym of ***cattle trucking.***

BOZD
Acronym of ***back optic zone diameter.***

BOZR
Acronym of ***back optic zone radius.***

BPR
Acronym of back peripheral radius.

brachytherapy
Locally applied radiotherapy. A radioactive source is placed next to the tumour.

bradycardia
Reduced heart rate.

brain mapping
Technique in which lots of electrodes are used to record multiple **visual evoked potentials**, to give location of activity. The reference is the mean of all the recordings.

brain stem
Lower part of the brain. Adjoins to and is structurally continuous with the spinal cord.

Braley's sign
Increased **intraocular pressure** in **elevation**, seen in **thyroid eye disease.**

branch retinal vein occlusion
A **retinal vein occlusion** only affecting one branch of the retinal vein. Typically occurs in the superior-temporal **fundus.** *Acronym is BRVO.*

BRAO
Acronym of branch ***retinal artery occlusion.***

break point
Synonym of ***fusional vergence.***

bright field magnifier
A dome or **bar magnifier** that provides an undistorted image over the surface. *Synonym is* ***flat field magnifier.***

Broca–Sulzer effect
Very brief flashes of light appear brighter than they actually are.

Brodmann area 17
Synonym of ***primary visual cortex.***

brolene
Synonym of ***propamidine.***

Brown's syndrome
Condition in which the **superior oblique** tendon has mechanically restricted movement through the **trochlea** and therefore cannot fully relax. Causes a restriction of **elevation** in **adduction** (sometimes with up/downshoot), and appears clinically similar to an **inferior oblique** underaction (differentiate by **forced duction test**). Can be either congenital or acquired. May be **hypotropia** in **primary position**. *Synonyms are **Brown's tendon sheath syndrome** and **superior oblique tendon sheath syndrome**.*

Brown's tendon sheath syndrome
*Synonym of **Brown's syndrome**.*

Bruch's membrane
The membrane between the **retinal pigment epithelium** and the **choriocapillaris**. Has five sublayers: retinal pigment epithelium membrane; collagen; elastic fibre mesh; collagen; choriocapillaris basement membrane.

Brückner test
Assessment of the **pupil**, **corneal**, and **fundus** reflexes from a distance, with a direct **ophthalmoscope**. Used as a quick, minimally invasive method of screening for **strabismus**, pupil defects, high refractive error, and **media opacity** in children.

brunescent cataract
A **cataract** with a brown appearance.

Bruns' nystagmus
Nystagmus caused by a tumour of the cerebellopontine angle. A high amplitude, low frequency nystagmus is seen when looking towards the side of the head with the lesion, and low amplitude, high frequency nystagmus is seen when looking contralaterally to the lesion.

Brushfield spots
White/grey spots on the iris, not uncommon in children, and very common in **Down syndrome**. They are due to accumulation of connective tissue.

BRVO
*Acronym of **branch retinal vein occlusion**.*

BSP
Acronym of back surface power.

BSV
Acronym of binocular single vision.

BU
Acronym of base up.

bulbar
Of the **globe**(s).

bulbar conjunctiva
The exposed part of the **conjunctiva** covering the **sclera**.

bulbar conjunctival hyperaemia
A complication of contact lens wear; redness of the **conjunctiva** with many causes, such as dry eye, allergy, poor lens fit, etc.

bulbar sheath
Synonym of ***Tenon's capsule.***

bull's eye maculopathy
Retinal pigment degeneration at **macula**, causing a concentric ring appearance. A sign of **oedema** or degeneration of the retina.

bulla
Fluid-filled blister found in severe **corneal oedema**. Causes reduced **visual acuity** and pain on rupturing. *Plural is* ***bullae.***

bullae
Plural of ***bulla.***

bullous keratopathy
Chronic **corneal oedema** with **blebs/bullae** caused by depletion of **corneal endothelium** cells. Painful.

Bunsen–Roscoe–Bloch law
Synonym of ***Bloch's law.***

buphthalmia
Synonym of ***buphthalmos.***

buphthalmos
Enlarged eye and **cornea** due to high **intraocular pressure** in early development, usually causing infantile **glaucoma**. Hazy cornea and blue **sclera**. *Synonyms are* ***buphthalmia*** *and* ***hydrophthalmos.***

Burian–Allen contact lens electrode
A bipolar **scleral contact lens** (has reference and active electrodes incorporated). Requires anaesthetic.

Burton lamp
An ultraviolet lamp (~350 nm) with magnifying glass sometimes used in contact lens fitting.

BUT
Acronym of ***tear breakup time.***

button
In fused bifocals, the piece that is added to the **contact curve** (the **addition**).

button curve
The curve of a fused bifocal into which the **button** is placed. ~0.25 D steeper than the **contact curve** to prevent trapped air.

button lenticular
A positive **lenticular lens**.

BV
Acronym of binocular vision.

BVA
Acronym of binocular vision anomaly.

BVD
Acronym of ***back vertex distance****.*

BVP
Acronym of ***back vertex power****.*

C

c
Abbreviation of con (with).

c-wave
Wave in **electroretinography**; only seen following **dark adaptation**, due to reduction in potassium ions from closure of photoreceptor outer segment cation channels.

C/I
Abbreviation of contraindication.

C/O
Acronym of complains of.

CA
*Acronym of **chromatic aberration**.*

CAB
Acronym of cellulose acetate butyrate.

CAEL
Acronym of constant axial edge lift.

CAI
Acronym of carbonic anhydrase inhibitor.

calcific emboli
Single, white emboli of the **fundus** vessels found close to the **optic disc.** Cause permanent obstruction.

caloric testing
Irrigation of the external meatus. The difference in temperature between the liquid and body creates a convection current in the horizontal **semicircular canal**, stimulating the **kinocilia,** resulting in **vestibulo-ocular reflex nystagmus**.

CALT
*Acronym of **conjunctival-associated lymphoid tissue**.*

CAM
Acronym of cell adhesion molecule.

C

Campbell effect
Explanation for poor **visual acuity** in the peripheral retina due to, in combination; the **Stiles–Crawford effect**, the arrangement of the photoreceptor array, and peripheral lens **aberrations**.

campimetry
Perimetry of the central **visual field** only.

canal of Cloquet
Synonym of ***Cloquet's canal.***

canal of Hannover
Synonym of ***Hannover's canal.***

canal of Petit
Synonym of ***Petit's canal.***

canal of Schlemm
Synonym of ***Schlemm's canal.***

canal of Stilling
Synonym of ***hyaloid artery.***

canaliculi
Tubes leading from the **puncta**; drain tears into the **lacrimal sac**. *Singular is* ***canaliculus.***

canaliculitis
Inflammation of the **canaliculus**.

canaliculus
Singular of ***canaliculi.***

candela
Measure of luminous power in a given direction. *Abbreviation is* ***cd.***

candidiasis
Infection by candida yeast. Can occur in the retina. *Synonym is* ***thrush.***

canthi
Plural of ***canthus.***

canthus
The 'corners' of the external eye, where the **conjunctiva** folds and the **eyelids** begin. *Plural is* ***canthi.***

Capgras delusion
Psychiatric disorder characterised by the belief that friends and relatives have been replaced by imposters. Believed to result from disconnection between the **inferotemporal cortex** and the limbic system.

capillary haemangioma
Common **benign tumour** appearing shortly after birth, often on the upper **eyelid**. Most spontaneously resolve. *Synonym is* ***strawberry naevus****.*

capsaicin drops
Drops of dilute chilli. Used as a chemical means of determining **corneal touch threshold**.

capsular bag
Synonym of ***lens capsule****.*

capsular fibrosis
A rare type of **posterior capsular opacification**; usually occurs up to 6 months post-**cataract** surgery, due to **capsular phimosis**.

capsular phimosis
Contraction of the **lens capsule**.

capsule
Synonym of ***lens capsule****.*

capsulorhexis
Surgical removal of part of the **lens capsule**, such as during **cataract** surgery. *Synonym is* ***capsulorrhexis****.*

capsulorrhexis
Synonym of ***capsulorhexis****.*

capsulotomy
Procedure in which a hole is made in the **lens capsule** with a **yttrium aluminium garnet laser**, usually to treat **posterior capsular opacification**.

captive bubble method
Method of measuring the **wetting angle** of a contact lens; the lens is submerged, and a gas bubble is floated up to the contact lens in solution. The angle the bubble forms with the lens is measured – this is the wetting angle.

carcinoma
Cancer of epithelial cells.

carcinoma in situ
A **carcinoma** that has not yet spread to other tissues.

C

carotenoid
A class of organic pigments ranging from yellow to red. Can contribute to lung cancer in smokers.

carotid endarterectomy
Surgical removal of deposits on the inside of the carotid. Helps to prevent **stroke**.

catadioptrics
Optical term referring to reflections & reflectors and **refraction** & refractors, when used in a single system.

cataract
An opacity of the crystalline lens. *Synonyms are* ***lens opacity*** *and* ***lenticular opacity****.*

catoptrics
Optical term referring to reflections and reflectors.

cattle trucking
The appearance of occasional patches of blood in inactive blood vessels. *Synonym is* ***box-carring****.*

caudal
Posterior.

caudal central subdivision
Portion of the **oculomotor nerve** nucleus that supplies the **levator palpebrae superioris**.

caustic
The envelope of light rays reflected or refracted by a curved surface.

cavernous haemangioma
Orbital tumour with onset in the 4th–5th decades of life. Usually just behind the **globe**. May cause **choroidal folds**.

CCF
Acronym of carotico-cavernous fistula.

CCT
Acronym of ***central corneal thickness****.*

CCTV magnifier
Synonym of ***video magnifier****.*

cd
Abbreviation of ***candela****.*

CD
Acronym of centration distance.

CDK
Acronym of ***climatic droplet keratopathy****.*

CE
Acronym of cataract extraction/Conformité Européenne.

cellophane maculopathy
Mild form of **epiretinal membrane**.

cells and flare
White blood cells and protein leaked into the **anterior chamber**. Seen in inflammatory conditions with the use of a slit lamp using a conical beam of light.

cellulitis
Inflamed soft tissue.

cemented bifocal
Bifocal in which the **addition** segment is a separate piece of glass, stuck on with **epoxy resin**. Often placed on the front surface for **myopes**, and the back for **hyperopes**; there is a safety concern with placing the segment on the back, as this can cause injury if it becomes loose.

centrad
A rarely used unit of angular measure. 1 centrad = a deviation of 1 cm at a distance of 1 m.

central areolar choroidal dystrophy
Similar to **gyrate atrophy** but starts in the central retina instead of mid-periphery.

central corneal thickness
The thickness of the **cornea**, measured in microns by **pachymetry**. *Acronym is CCT.*

central nystagmus
Any **nystagmus** not related to the vestibular system (i.e. nystagmus that cannot be described as **peripheral nystagmus**).

central retinal artery
Branches from the ophthalmic artery, enters the **optic nerve** ~1 cm behind eye, climbs the nasal cup. *Acronym is* ***CRA****.*

central retinal vein occlusion
A **retinal vein occlusion** affecting the entire retinal vein. *Acronym is* ***CRVO****.*

central serous chorioretinopathy
Synonym of ***central serous retinopathy****.*

central serous choroidopathy
Synonym of ***central serous retinopathy.***

central serous retinopathy
Idiopathic condition usually found in young males under stress, or pregnant women. The **macula** becomes raised due to leakage of fluid from the **choriocapillaris** into the **retinal pigment epithelium**. This causes a slight hyperopic shift and **metamorphopsia**. Usually the condition resolves spontaneously. *Acronym is* ***CSR****. Synonyms are* ***central serous chorioretinopathy****,* ***central serous choroidopathy****, and* ***idiopathic central serous retinopathy****.*

centre of rotation condition
Rule used by dispensing opticians in lens design: for every 1° of **pantoscopic tilt**, lower the **optical centre** by 1 mm.

centre-surround antagonism
The situation in which a **receptive field** is surrounded by an antagonistic receptive field, as seen in the retina.

centrocaecal field defect
A paracentral **visual field** defect that encompasses the blind spot.

cephalalgia
Headache.

cerebral achromatopsia
Achromatopsia following damage to **V4**. Much rarer than **cerebral dyschromatopsia**. *Synonym is* ***colour agnosia****.*

cerebral akinetopsia
Synonym of ***akinetopsia****.*

cerebral dyschromatopsia
Desaturation of colour perception following damage to **V4**.

cerebral palsy
Permanent, non-progressive disorder of movement and posture. Whilst many affected individuals have learning difficulties, some may have no learning difficulty at all. **Cerebral visual impairment** may or may not be present.

cerebral visual impairment
Umbrella term used to describe perceptual problems following diffuse brain damage, particularly in patients with **cerebral palsy**. *Synonym is* ***cortical visual impairment****.*

CF
Acronym of counting fingers.

CFF
Acronym of ***critical flicker fusion frequency****.*

cGMP
Acronym of cyclic guanosine monophosphate.

chalazion
Non-infective obstruction and **inflammation** of **meibomian gland**s or **Zeis glands**. Larger than a **stye**. Painless unless pressing on eye. *Synonym is **meibomian gland granuloma**.*

chalcosis
Copper deposits in tissue.

Chandler syndrome
Corneal oedema seen in **iridocorneal endothelial syndrome.**

change blindness
Normal phenomenon which dictates that we find it very difficult to discern a change in the visual scene if the change occurs during a transient interruption of the image, such as during a blink.

channels of Sondermann
Collecting ducts leading to **Schlemm's canal**. Collect **aqueous humour**.

Charles Bonnet syndrome
Visual **hallucination**s caused by **low vision**. Sufferers are always aware that the hallucinations are not real.

Chédiak–Higashi syndrome
Rare genetic disorder. Causes **oculocutaneous albinism**.

chemical shift imaging
*Synonym of **magnetic resonance spectroscopy**.*

chemosis
Conjunctival oedema.

cherry-red spot
The appearance of the **choroid** through the **macula** during **oedema**. A sign of many conditions, including **retinal artery occlusion**.

Chiari malformation
*Synonym of **Arnold–Chiari malformation**.*

chiasm
*Synonym of **optic chiasm**.*

chiasmal pupil
Poor reaction to light in the temporal **visual fields**. Possible sign of a pituitary tumour.

C

CHL
*Acronym of **chloramphenicol**.*

chlamydia psittaci
A pathogen that causes **trachoma**.

chlamydia trachomatis
A pathogen that causes **trachoma**.

chlamydial conjunctivitis
Causes mucopurulence with a follicular appearance and a peripheral **keratitis**. There are two major types: **trachoma** and **inclusion conjunctivitis**.

chloramphenicol
A mild broad spectrum antibiotic, routinely used by **optometrist**s. Not effective against **pseudomonas**. **ADR**s include aplastic aenemia and grey baby syndrome. *Acronym is **CHL**.*

chlorolabe
The pigment present in **M-cone**s.

chloropsia
Green **chromatopsia**.

chloroquine
An anti-malarial drug. Long term use may cause **chloroquine retinopathy**.

chloroquine retinopathy
Parafoveal atrophy, reduced **visual acuity**, blue-yellow colour vision defects, and **protanomaly**. Caused by prolonged **chloroquine** or **hydroxychloroquine** use.

cholesterol emboli
*Synonym of **Hollenhorst plaque**.*

choriocapillaris
Layer of capillaries in the **choroid**, located between **Sattler's layer** and **Bruch's membrane**.

chorioid
*Synonym of **choroid**.*

chorioretinitis
Simultaneous **inflammation** of both the **choroid** and retina.

choroid
Part of the **uvea** lying between the retina and **sclera**. Contains a vascular network supplying the outer retina. Composed of four layers: **Haller's layer**, **Sattler's layer**, the **choriocapillaris**, and **Bruch's membrane**. *Synonym is **chorioid**.*

C

choroidal folds
Folds in the **fundus** that suggests something is pressing on the **globe** or that **intraocular pressure** is very low. Usually seen as horizontal folds.

choroidal haemangioma
A rare **benign tumour**. Causes an elevated patch near the **posterior pole** with an orange-red appearance. May cause a **retinal detachment**.

choroidal naevus
A **benign tumour** of the **choroid**. Will increase in size in puberty, shouldn't thereafter.

choroidal neovascular membrane
Neovascularisation from the **choroid** into the retina in response to **hypoxia**. A network of vessels with the potential to leak fluid and blood. *Synonyms are* ***choroidal neovascularisation*** *and* ***subretinal neovascular membrane****.*

choroidal neovascularisation
Synonym of ***choroidal neovascular membrane****.*

choroidal pneumocystosis
A rare infection of the **fundus** associated with **AIDS**.

choroideraemia
An X-linked retinal pigment dysfunction, causing distinctly patchy **retinal pigment epithelium** and **choroid**al atrophy. Patients experience **nyctalopia**.

choroiditis
Inflammation of the **choroid**.

CHP
Acronym of ***compensatory head posture****.*

Christmas tree cataract
A **lens opacity** with a sparkling appearance. Can be caused by **myotonic dystrophy**.

chromatic aberration
Measure of the angle of dispersion of a prism. Causes images to form with coloured fringes. *Acronym is* ***CA****.*

chromatophene
Perception of coloured rings or halos, as a **hallucination**, e.g. due to **classic migraine**.

chromatopsia
Excessively saturated colour perception, e.g. due to recent removal of **cataract** or **hallucination**. Specific forms are **chloropsia**, **cyanopsia**, **erythropsia**, and **xanthopsia**.

chronic open angle glaucoma
Refers to **primary open angle glaucoma** or **pigmentary glaucoma**. *Acronym is* ***COAG***.

CHRPE
Acronym of ***congenital hypertrophy of the retinal pigment epithelium***.

CI
Acronym of ***convergence insufficiency***.

cilia
The hairs that grow at the **palpebral** margins. *Singular is* ***cilium***. *Synonyms are* ***eyelashes*** *and* ***lash***.

ciliary body
Collectively refers to the **ciliary muscle** and **ciliary processes**.

ciliary ganglion
Located in the **orbit**; receives axons from the **Edinger–Westphal nucleus**. Innervates the **ciliary muscle** and **sphincter pupillae**.

ciliary margin
The margin between iris and **ciliary body**. *Synonym is* ***iris root***.

ciliary muscle
Produces **aqueous humour** and is attached to the **Zonules of Zinn**. Contraction causes **accommodation**.

ciliary muscle tonus allowance
Even when **accommodation** is relaxed, there is still some muscle tonus in the **ciliary muscle**. During **cycloplegic** refraction, some of this is relaxed. Tonus allowance is the power that allows for over-relaxation during cycloplegic **refraction** such that the final result is not over-plussed.

ciliary processes
The ridges of the **pars plicata**. Connected to the **zonules of Zinn**. *Synonym is* ***corona ciliaris***.

cilio-spinal centre of Budge
Part of the sympathetic **pupil** pathway. Receives signals from the posterior hypothalamus and projects to the superior cervical ganglion.

cilioretinal artery
A blood vessel emergent from the temporal **optic disc**, providing an extra blood supply to inner retina between the **macula** and **optic nerve head**. This is found in ~30% of people.

cilium
Singular of ***cilia***.

circle of least confusion
In an astigmatic **pencil** of light, the exact point midway between the two principle meridians' **focal points**; giving the best possible, but inevitably out of focus, image.

circle of Zinn
*Synonym of **circle of Zinn–Haller**.*

circle of Zinn–Haller
Anastomosing ring of arteries around the **annulus of Zinn**. *Synonym is **circle of Zinn**.*

circus senilis
Arcus senilis when it extends to a full circle.

CJD
Acronym of Creutzfeldt–Jakob disease.

CK
*Acronym of conductive **keratoplasty**.*

CL
Acronym of contact lens.

CLAPC
*Acronym of **contact lens associated papillary conjunctivitis**.*

CLARE
*Acronym of **contact lens induced acute red eye**.*

classic choroidal neovascularisation
Choroidal neovascularisation in which the **choroidal neovascular membrane** is above the **retinal pigment epithelium** and shows up easily on **fluorescein angiography**.

classic migraine
Migraine with a **migraine aura**.

classical psychophysical methods
Psychophysical methods for estimating perceptual thresholds. Includes the **method of adjustment, method of constant stimuli**, and **method of limits**.

clear lens exchange
*Synonym of **refractive lens exchange**.*

CLEB
*Acronym of **contact lens associated endothelial bedewing**.*

CLIDE
Acronym of contact lens induced dry eye.

C

climatic droplet keratopathy
Synonym of ***spheroidal degeneration.***

CLIPC
Acronym of ***contact lens induced papillary conjunctivitis.***

Cloquet's canal
The remnant of the **hyaloid vessel** and **primary vitreous**. Apparent as an antero-posterior canal through the **vitreous humour** in normal individuals. *Synonym is* ***canal of Cloquet.***

closed angle glaucoma
Damage occurring to the **optic nerve head** due to increased pressure in the eye due to partial or complete obstruction of the **anterior chamber angle**. *Synonym is* ***angle closure glaucoma.***

closed globe
An eye without a full-thickness wound.

clover-leaf field
An automated **perimetry** printout showing a 'clover leaf' shape due to fatigue effect after successfully seeing the first few stimuli; some **visual field** screening programmes begin with these stimuli locations.

CLPC
Acronym of ***contact lens induced papillary conjunctivitis.***

CLPU
Acronym of ***contact lens induced peripheral ulcer.***

CLSLK
Acronym of ***contact lens induced superior limbic keratoconjunctivitis.***

CMO
Acronym of ***cystoid macular oedema.***

CMV
Acronym of ***cytomegalovirus.***

CN
Acronym of cranial nerve.

CNPU
Acronym of ***culture negative peripheral ulcer.***

CNS
Acronym of central nervous system.

CNV
*Acronym of **choroidal neovascularisation**.*

COAG
*Acronym of **chronic open angle glaucoma**.*

Coats' disease
Exudative retinal disease. Causes **leukocoria**, **strabismus**, **aneurysms**, and **telangiectasia**. Can cause **serous retinal detachment**.

Coats' white ring
Scar left on the **cornea** after removal of a foreign body.

cobblestone degeneration
*Synonym of **progressive chorioretinal atrophy**.*

cobblestone retinopathy
*Synonym of **progressive chorioretinal atrophy**.*

Cochet–Bonnet aesthesiometer
A type of **aesthesiometer** that measures **corneal touch threshold** using different lengths of nylon. Corneal touch threshold is defined at the length of nylon that is felt by the patient on 50% of applications to the **cornea**.

Cogan–Reese syndrome
Diffuse iris **naevus** with pigmented nodules seen in **iridocorneal endothelial syndrome**.

Cogan's apraxia
*Synonym of **saccade initiation failure**.*

Cogan's lid twitch
Movement from **depression** to **primary position** causes **eyelid** to **twitch** up and overshoot before settling.

Cogan's microcystic dystrophy
Non-progressive **corneal epithelium** dystrophy with the appearance of 'maps', dots, 'fingerprints', and cysts. May cause **corneal erosion**s or mild discomfort, or patients may be asymptomatic. Often **bilateral**. Non-familial. *Synonyms are **anterior basement membrane dystrophy, epithelial basement membrane dystrophy, fingerprint dystrophy**, and **map-dot-fingerprint dystrophy**.*

Cohen syndrome
Rare genetic disorder that can cause high **myopia**.

coherent
Describes light which is in-phase.

collagen cross-linking
Procedure used to strengthen the **corneal stroma** in **keratoconus**. Riboflavin is activated by ultraviolet light. *Synonym is **corneal cross-linking**.*

collarette
1. The ridge of the iris, which divides the pupillary and ciliary zones where the **sphincter pupillae** and **dilator pupillae** overlap.
2. Crusts around the base of the **cilia**.

collateral
A blood vessel that has swollen in an attempt to drain blood. Can occur following a **retinal vein occlusion**.

Collier's sign
Eyelid retraction, indicative of a midbrain **lesion**, such as **dorsal midbrain syndrome**.

coloboma
A hole in one of the structures of the eye, caused by the **choroid**al fissure not closing properly during embryological development.

colour after-effect
Long exposure to a colour bleaches photoreceptors, causing false colour to be perceived.

colour agnosia
*Synonym of **cerebral achromatopsia**.*

colour anomia
Inability to name colours, despite being able to recognise them.

colour blindness
*Synonym of **achromatopsia**.*

colour constancy
The fact that colours are perceived approximately the same under different levels of **illumination**. (This concept fails with narrow band lighting.)

colour deficiency
*Synonym of **dyschromatopsia**.*

colour rendering
Similarity between an image and object's colours.

colour rendering index
How well a surface's reflections are colour rendered. Scale from 0 to 100 (100 = perfect).

colour temperature
The required temperature of a **black body** such that it emits a given colour.

coma
A spherical higher-order **aberration** experienced by off-**axis** point sources.

comfort bridge
A large spectacle bridge providing support over the whole nose. *Synonyms are **anatomical bridge** and **saddle bridge**.*

comitance
Condition in which the angle between the eyes (whether this be strabismic or orthophoric) is maintained in all positions of **gaze**. *Synonym is **concomitance**.*

common migraine
Migraine without a **migraine aura**.

common tendinous ring
*Synonym of **annulus of Zinn**.*

commotio retinae
Milky appearance to the retina following blunt trauma due to neuro-retinal damage.

compensatory eye movement
Eye movement intending to maintain a stable image on the retina.

compensatory head posture
*Synonym of **abnormal head posture**.*

complementary colours
Colours which can be combined, in light form, to form white. These colour pairs also cause each other's **afterimage** if shone on the retina; e.g. blue and yellow; red and cyan; green and purple.

complete monochromatism
*Synonym of **rod monochromatism**.*

complex cell
Type of cell found in the **primary visual cortex** (**V1**), **V2**, and **V3**, with **receptive fields** that detect motion of oriented edges. Do not code absolute location, only the presence or absence of the stimulus.

compound hyperopic astigmatism
Astigmatism in which the whole astigmatic cone falls behind the retina.

compound myopic astigmatism
Astigmatism in which the whole astigmatic cone falls in front of the retina.

COMT
Acronym of catechol-O-methyl transferase.

concomitance
*Synonym of **comitance**.*

concretion
Small hard white calcium spots found on the **tarsal conjunctiva**. Patients are usually asymptomatic. Can be removed with a needle.

conditioning flash
The first flash presented in **electroretinography**: unrecorded, as it simply habituates the patient to the flashes.

cone monochromat
An individual who has rods and only one type of cone.

confocal
Having the same **focal point**.

confusion
The perception of two images that cannot fuse.

congenital
Describes any condition which is present at birth.

congenital choroidal hypertrophy
*Synonym of **congenital hypertrophy of the retinal pigment epithelium**.*

congenital hypertrophy of the retinal pigment epithelium
Sharply demarcated brown to black **lesion** at the **fundus**; darker than a **naevus** or **melanoma**, due to thickening of the **retinal pigment epithelium** and photoreceptor loss. Causes a **visual field** defect. Usually grows very slowly. *Acronym is **CHRPE**. Synonym is **congenital choroidal hypertrophy**.*

congenital idiopathic nystagmus
*Synonym of **idiopathic infantile nystagmus**.*

congenital nystagmus
*Synonym of **infantile nystagmus**.*

congenital stationary nightblindness
Group of conditions causing **nyctalopia**. There are four subtypes: **congenital stationary nightblindness type I sub-type A**, **congenital stationary nightblindness type I sub-type B**, **congenital stationary nightblindness type II**, and **congenital stationary nightblindness type III**. *Acronym is **CSNB**.*

congenital stationary nightblindness type I sub-type A
Characterised by a normal **fundus** appearance but abnormal photoreceptor inner segments. **a-wave** and **b-wave** of **electroretinography** are abnormal.

congenital stationary nightblindness type I sub-type B
Characterised by a normal **fundus** appearance but abnormal **inner plexiform layer.** No **b-wave** on **electroretinography**.

congenital stationary nightblindness type II
Characterised by abnormal **fundus**. Caused by either **fundus albipunctatus** or **Oguchi's disease**.

congenital stationary nightblindness type III
X-linked recessive condition. **Myopia, nystagmus**, and **low vision**. Rod **electroretinography** has no **b-wave**.

congenital strabismus syndrome
Synonym of ***infantile esotropia syndrome.***

congruous
Having the same shape.

conjugate eye movement
Synonym of ***version.***

conjunctiva
Membrane covering the inner **eyelids** and anterior **sclera**. Comprises the **tarsal conjunctiva, fornix conjunctiva**, and **bulbar conjunctiva**.

conjunctival lymphoma
Tumour of the **conjunctival-associated lymphoid tissue**: appears as fleshy 'fish-like' sub-conjunctival mass.

conjunctival melanoma
Nodular. Malignant; may be nodules on **primary acquired melanosis**, or from **naevus**, etc.

conjunctival-associated lymphoid tissue
Mucosa-associated lymphoid tissue found in the **conjunctiva**. *Acronym is* ***CALT.***

conjunctivitis
Inflammation of the **conjunctiva**. Also known as 'pink eye'.

conjunctivochalasis
Excessive **lid-parallel conjunctival folds**, leading to symptoms of dry eye, irritation, **epiphora**, etc.

consecutive esotropia
An **esotropia** that was previously another type of **strabismus**. Grouped as either **spontaneous consecutive esotropia** or **post-operative consecutive esotropia.**

C

consecutive exotropia
An **exotropia** that was previously another type of **strabismus**. Grouped as either **spontaneous consecutive exotropia** or **post-operative consecutive exotropia**.

consensual pupillary reflex
Light shone into one eye causes constriction of the **pupil** in the fellow eye due to dual pretectal signalling.

constant axial edge lift lens
Describes the fit of a contact lens in which the clearance between the contact lens and the **cornea** is constant.

constant esotropia
An **esotropia** that is always present. The extent may vary with **accommodation** or not at all.

constant exotropia
An **exotropia** that is always present. Either early onset or decompensated intermittent exotropia.

constringence
The inverse of the dispersion value of a material. *Synonyms are* ***Abbe value*** *and* ***V number****.*

contact curve
In fused bifocals, the curve to which the **button** is added.

contact lens associated endothelial bedewing
Inflammatory response of the **corneal endothelium** caused by **hypoxia**. *Acronym is* ***CLEB****.*

contact lens associated papillary conjunctivitis
Synonym of ***contact lens induced papillary conjunctivitis****.*

contact lens induced acute red eye
Inflammatory response to extended wear of contact lenses. Causes **hyperaemia** and multiple **sterile corneal infiltrates**. *Acronyms are* ***ARE*** *and* ***CLARE****. Synonym is* ***tight lens syndrome****.*

contact lens induced papillary conjunctivitis
Allergic response related to contact lens wear/solution sensitivity. Causes **hyperaemia** and roughness under **eyelids**. *Acronyms are* ***CLIPC*** *and* ***CLPC****. Synonyms are* ***contact lens associated papillary conjunctivitis*** *and* ***papillary conjunctivitis****.*

contact lens induced peripheral ulcer
A single **sterile corneal infiltrate** <2 mm in size, usually found in the peripheral **cornea**. Caused by reaction to toxins released by **staphylococcus**. Stains with **fluorescein** and causes **conjunctival hyperaemia**, soreness, and lacrimation. Onset is usually acute. The **anterior chamber** is usually quiet. *Acronym is* ***CLPU****. Synonym is* ***culture negative peripheral ulcer****.*

contact lens induced superior limbic keratoconjunctivitis
Condition often caused by **thimerosal** hypersensitivity. *Acronym is* ***CLSLK****. Synonyms are* ***superior limbic keratoconjunctivitis*** *and* ***thimerosal keratopathy****.*

contact tonometer
Any **tonometer** that makes contact with the **cornea** in order to measure **intraocular pressure**. Most of these devices are **applanation tonometers**.

contour interaction
Describes the **crowding effect** induced by any line or contour adjacent to a visual target.

contraction furrows
Furrows formed at the back of the iris when the **pupil** dilates.

contracture
Contracted muscle that cannot relax fully.

contralateral
Anatomical term. Means 'on the opposite side'.

contralateral synergist
Extraocular muscle on the opposite side, achieving the same function. *Synonym is* ***yoke muscle****.*

contralesional
On the opposite hemisphere/**hemifield** as a brain **lesion**.

contrapulsion
Lateropulsion in which patients have **hypermetric saccades** in the **contralateral** direction of, and **hypometric saccades** in the **ipsilateral** direction of, a brain lesion. The opposite of **ipsipulsion**.

contrast
Difference in luminance between two parts of a scene (task and background). May be defined as **Weber contrast** or **Michelson contrast**.

contrast rendering factor
Indicates how local lighting will affect **contrast** compared to test conditions. *Acronym is CRF.*

contrast reserve
The ratio between the absolute **contrast** sensitivity of an individual to what they can comfortably see (for example, for extended reading). Usually 10:1.

contrast sensitivity
The ability to discern objects from other objects and backgrounds. *Acronym is* ***CS****.*

contrast sensitivity function
The **spatial modulation transfer function** of the visual system.

contrast threshold
The lowest **contrast** at which a target is detectable. *Synonym is **Weber's constant**.*

contraversion
An eye movement made in the opposite direction to a stimulus. Observed in the **antisaccade** task. *Adjective form is **contraversive**.*

contraversive
*Adjective form of **contraversion**.*

contrecoup injury
Brain damage situated at the opposite side of the head to a **coup injury**. Due to rapid deceleration of the brain, causing impact against the skull.

contusion
Bruise.

convergence
The opposite of **divergence**. In reference to light: describes a **pencil** of rays that is becoming more focused. In relation to the eyes: describes a **vergence** eye movement in which the angle between the visual axes decreases.

convergence accommodation
*Synonym of **vergence accommodation**.*

convergence amplitude
The maximum extent to which a patient's eyes can converge. Quantified as the **near point of convergence**.

convergence esotropia
*Synonym of **convergence excess**.*

convergence excess
Describes the condition in which a patient converges too much when viewing a near target. Binocular single vision is present when viewing in the distance but **esotropia** is present when accommodating for near **fixation**. *Synonym is **convergence esotropia**.*

convergence fusional reserve
*Synonym of **positive fusional reserve**.*

convergence insufficiency
Inability to obtain and/or maintain adequate **convergence** without undue effort. *Acronym is **CI**.*

convergence nystagmus
*Synonym of **convergence retraction saccadic pulses.***

convergence paralysis
Often due to rostral midbrain **lesion**. Medial recti don't **convergence**, but **versions** and **ductions** are normal.

convergence retraction nystagmus
*Synonym of **convergence retraction saccadic pulses.***

convergence retraction saccadic pulses
Saccadic pulses seen in **dorsal midbrain syndrome**; when attempting **convergence**, eyes shake forward and back in the **orbit**. *Synonyms are **convergence nystagmus, convergence retraction nystagmus,** and **convergence tremor of Elschnig.***

convergence tremor of Elschnig
*Synonym of **convergence retraction saccadic pulses.***

copper wiring
In **arteriosclerosis**, as vessels are infiltrated with **lipid** deposits, they resemble copper.

corectopia
Condition in which the **pupil** is not in the centre of the iris. *Synonym is **ectopic pupil.***

coredialysis
*Synonym of **iridodialysis.***

cornea
Transparent window at the front of the eye. Composed of six layers: the **corneal epithelium, Bowman's membrane**, the **corneal stroma, Dua's layer, Descemet's membrane**, and the **corneal endothelium**.

corneal arcus
*Synonym of **arcus senilis.***

corneal astigmatism
Astigmatism induced by inequal curvature of the **cornea**. Every 0.1 mm difference in **keratometry** readings accounts for approximately 0.50 DC of astigmatism.

corneal cap
The steepest part of the **cornea**, usually located slightly supero-nasally.

corneal cross-linking
*Synonym of **collagen cross-linking.***

corneal ectasia
Thinning of the **cornea**. *Synonym is **ectasia.***

C

corneal endothelium
The most posterior **cornea**l layer. Composed of a single layer of hexagonal cells that do not regenerate.

corneal epithelial basal cells
All epithelial cells begin as basal cells, turn into **corneal epithelial wing cells**, then **corneal epithelial squamous cells**.

corneal epithelial squamous cells
The last (most anterior) phase in the **corneal epithelium**, composed of **squamous** cells. Eventually the cells apoptose.

corneal epithelial wing cells
Formed from ageing **corneal epithelial basal cells**. Later become **corneal epithelial squamous cells**.

corneal epithelium
The most anterior layer of the **cornea**; approximately six cells thick. Composed of **corneal epithelial squamous cells, corneal epithelial wing cells**, and **corneal epithelial basal cells**.

corneal erosion
Epithelium sloughing off. *Synonym is **corneal melt**.*

corneal farinata
Flour-like deposits in the posterior **corneal stroma**, composed of **lipofuscin**. Normal age-related change. *Synonym is **farinata**.*

corneal fibrils
Found in the stroma. Have a uniform diameter to maintain transparency. Overlap of fibrils causes 'banding' effect.

corneal hysteresis
A property of the **cornea** measured by the **Ocular Response Analyser**; a measurement of the visco-elastic properties of the cornea related to the speed of recoil following **applanation**. Its clinical significance is unknown.

corneal lamellae
Produced by **keratocytes**. Extend between limbi. ~200 layers are found in the **cornea**.

corneal lens
*Synonym of **rigid gas permeable**.*

corneal melt
*Synonym of **corneal erosion**.*

corneal oedema
Swelling and haziness of the **corneal stroma** due to accumulation of fluid. Either acute (**hydrops**) or chronic (**bullous keratopathy**).

corneal reflex

1. Blink reflex stimulated by touching the **cornea.**
2. The outermost of the **Purkinje images** caused by the **corneal epithelium.** 100× brighter than the other Purkinje images.

corneal refractive therapy

Synonym of ***orthokeratology.***

corneal stroma

Thick layer of the **cornea** between **Bowman's membrane** and **Dua's layer**. Tough. More longitudinal collagen than lateral. *Synonym is* ***substantia propria.***

corneal touch threshold

How much force can be felt by the **cornea**. More sensitive towards the middle. Measured with an **aesthesiometer**. *Acronym is* ***CTT.***

corneal ulcer

An epithelial **abrasion** with a bacterial infection.

corneal verticillata

Pigment lines (deposits) on **cornea**, associated with the use of antipsychotics and antiarrhythmics. *Synonyms are* ***amiodarone keratopathy*** *and* ***vortex keratopathy.***

corneoretinal potential

The electrical potential difference between the cornea and retina, which is measured in **electro-oculography**.

cornified skin

The outermost layer of skin.

corollary discharge

Synonym of ***efference copy.***

corona ciliaris

Synonym of ***ciliary processes.***

coronal plane

The anatomical plane that runs from the left to the right of the body. *Synonym is* ***frontal plane.***

corpora quadrigemina

The four colliculi in the mesencephalon.

corpus callosum

The white matter that connects the two halves of the brain.

corrected pattern standard deviation
In **visual field** testing, the **pattern standard deviation** with the effect of **short-term fluctuation** removed. Not available with the **Swedish interactive threshold algorithm**. Measured in decibels. *Acronym is* ***CPSD.***

cortical
In the cortex. May refer to the **visual cortex**.

cortical blindness
Blindness due to **lesion** or abnormality of the **visual cortex**; not primarily any other part of the visual pathway.

cortical eye fields
Collective term for the **frontal eye fields**, **supplemental eye fields**, and parietal eye fields.

cortical magnification
The fact that a greater area of **primary visual cortex** is devoted to **foveal** vision, and also a greater area for each foveal **ganglion cell** than other ganglion cells.

cortical visual impairment
Synonym of ***cerebral visual impairment.***

corticosteroid
Group of steroid hormones produced by adrenal cortex, often used as anti-inflammatories.

cosmetic contact lens
A contact lens that changes the appearance of the eye; may also provide refractive correction.

cosmetic shell
A **cosmetic contact lens** that is usually not transparent – used to mask unsightly ocular conditions.

cotton thread test
Synonym of ***phenol red test.***

cotton wool spots
Swelling of retinal nerve fibres due to local **ischaemia** and impaired axoplasmic flow. *Synonym is* ***soft exudates.***

couching
Primitive form of **cataract** surgery, in which a needle inserted into the eye is intended to displace a mature cataract into the **vitreous humour**.

coulometric technique
International standard for measuring Dk of **rigid gas permeable** contact lenses with Dk > 100.

coup injury
Brain damage situated at the site of impact of the head. Contrast with **contrecoup injury**.

covert attention
Visual attention on an object not in the **fovea**'s line of sight.

CP
Acronym of ***cerebral palsy****/colour perception.*

cpd
Acronym of cycles per degree.

CPSD
Acronym of ***corrected pattern standard deviation****.*

CR39
Abbreviation of Columbia resin 39.

CRA
Acronym of ***central retinal artery****.*

CRAO
Acronym of ***central retinal artery*** *occlusion.*

CRE
Acronym of corrected refractive error.

CRF
Acronym of ***contrast rendering factor****.*

crispening effect
Stimuli with intensity close to the background intensity appear to have unusually higher intensity contrast.

critical angle
The angle light must travel into a material such that total internal reflection occurs. Is defined as the sine of the inverse of the **refractive index** of the material.

critical duration
The longest period over which **temporal summation** can take place.

critical flicker frequency
Synonym of ***critical flicker fusion frequency****.*

critical flicker fusion frequency
Highest flicker rate detectable (at any **contrast**) or lowest detectable (in this case 'flicker' could refer to, for example, the transition between day and night). *Acronym is **CFF**. Synonyms are **critical flicker frequency** and **flicker fusion test**.*

critical period
*Synonym of **plastic period**.*

crocodile shagreen
Crocodile skin appearance to the **cornea**. Due to degeneration.

crocodile tears
Nerve fibres meant for salivatory gland project to the **lacrimal gland. Lacrimation** upon seeing food. Can occur due to aberrant regeneration of the facial nerve following **Bell's palsy**.

cross curve
In an ophthalmic lens, the difference between the cross curve and **base curve** = lens cylinder power.

cross cylinder
*Synonym of **Jackson cross cylinder**.*

crossed diplopia
*Synonym of **heteronymous diplopia**.*

crossed extensor reflex
A withdrawal reflex whereby one half of the body responds to support the other half.

crossed retinal disparity
Occurs in front of the **horopter**. **Diplopia** occurs outside **Panum's fusional area**. *Synonyms are **heteronymous retinal disparity**, **positive retinal disparity**, and **temporal retinal disparity**.*

Crouzon syndrome
Condition in which a shallow **orbit** causes **proptosis**. Often **exotropia**.

crowded disc
Describes a non-pathological **optic nerve head** with features that are hard to distinguish due to an excess of vessels in the area, perhaps due to a small **disc** size and closely packed nerve fibres.

crowding effect
The concept that objects are easier to see if not surrounded (applies to Snellen chart). *Synonym is **separation difficulty**.*

CRT
Acronym of cathode ray tube.

CRVO
Acronym of ***central retinal vein occlusion.***

CS
Acronym of ***contrast sensitivity.***

CSCR
Acronym of ***central serous chorioretinopathy.***

CSF
*Acronym of cerebrospinal fluid/****contrast sensitivity function.***

CSLO
Acronym of confocal scanning laser ***ophthalmoscope.***

CSMO
Acronym of clinically significant macular ***oedema.***

CSNB
Acronym of ***congenital stationary nightblindness.***

CSR
Acronym of ***central serous retinopathy.***

CT
Acronym of centre thickness/computed tomography/cover test.

CTT
Acronym of ***corneal touch threshold.***

culture negative peripheral ulcer
Synonym of ***contact lens induced peripheral ulcer.***

cuneate
Wedge shaped. Sometimes used to describe the nasal fibres of the **optic nerve head**.

Cushing syndrome
Endocrine pathology causing moon face, obesity, diabetes, and **hypertension**.

cutaneous horn
A keratinous skin lesion that appears as a horn. Typically develops slowly; may indicate malignancy.

cuticular drusen
Thickening of the basement membrane of the **retinal pigment epithelium**. *Synonym is* ***basal laminar drusen.***

CV
Acronym of colour vision.

CVA
Acronym of cerebrovascular accident.

CVE
Acronym of cerebrovascular event.

CVI
Acronym of ***cerebral visual impairment****/certificate of visual impairment.*

CXL
Acronym of ***collagen cross-linking/corneal cross-linking****.*

cyanolabe
The photosensitive pigment present in **S-cone**s.

cyanopsia
Blue **chromatopsia**. Often occurs for a period of time following **cataract** removal.

CYC
Abbreviation of ***cyclopentolate****.*

cyclectomy
Removal of part of the **ciliary body**.

cyclic esotropia
An **esotropia** that manifests on alternate days (or another given time period).

cyclitis
Inflammation of the **ciliary body**.

cyclodiode laser treatment
Treatment for advanced/difficult to treat **glaucoma**. Burns made to **ciliary body**, to decrease **aqueous humour** production.

cyclopean eye concept
The world is effectively seen as if through a single eye due to binocularity.

cyclopentolate
An antimuscarinic **cycloplegic**, routinely used by **optometrist**s. Typically available in 0.5% and 1% concentrations. *Abbreviation is* ***CYC****.*

cyclopia
Congenital disorder in which only one eye forms. Affected foetuses usually end in miscarriage or are stillborn. Can be caused by a mutation in **Sonic hedgehog homologue**.

cycloplegia
Paralysis of ciliary muscles, resulting in loss of **accommodation**.

cycloplegic
Any chemical that causes **cycloplegia**.

cyl
Abbreviation of cylinder.

cystoid diabetic maculopathy
*Synonym of **diffuse diabetic maculopathy**.*

cystoid macular oedema
Macular oedema accompanied with the development of painless cyst-like swelling. Fluid is found in the **outer plexiform layer**. Often presents 4–6 weeks after **cataract** surgery. *Acronym is **CMO**.*

cytochrome oxidase
Used to stain tissues. In **V1**, stains **blobs**; in **V2**, stains **stripes**.

cytokine
Protein family. Used to transmit messages between cells (often immune response).

cytokine tests
A test of the tears, measuring inflammatory response.

cytomegalovirus
A virus in the herpes family. Causes **cytomegalovirus retinitis** in the immuno-compromised. *Acronym is **CMV**.*

cytomegalovirus retinitis
Peripheral areas of white necrosis and haemorrhaging in the **fundus**.

cytotoxicity
Toxic to cells.

D

D
Abbreviation of ***dioptre****.*

d-wave
Wave in **electroretinography** to OFF-**bipolar cells**; occurs when a light is turned off after a time of **light adaptation**.

dacryoadenitis
Inflammation of **lacrimal glands**. Upper **eyelid** swells. Can be caused by infection/mumps.

dacryocystitis
Inflammation of the **nasolacrimal duct**.

dacryocystorhinostomy
Surgical procedure in which a new tear duct is created by removing a piece of the nose bone. A temporary tube prevents healing over. *Acronym is* ***DCR****.*

DALK
Acronym of ***deep anterior lamellar keratoplasty****.*

Dalrymple's sign
Eyelid retraction when viewing in the **primary position** due to **proptosis**. Causes **Kocher's sign**.

Daltonism
Synonym of ***achromatopsia****.*

dark adaptation
Synonym of ***adaptation****.*

datum line
The horizontal centre line of an ophthalmic lens.

Dawson, Trick, Litzkow electrode
Electrode consisting of a nylon fibre which is placed in the lower **fornix**. *Acronym is* ***DTL****.*

DC
Acronym of dioptres of cylinder.

DCR
Acronym of ***dacryocystorhinostomy****.*

DD
Acronym of disc diameters.

DDT
*Acronym of **dye disappearance test**.*

dDx
Abbreviation of differential diagnosis.

de Morsier syndrome
*Synonym of **septo-optic dysplasia**.*

de Vries–Rose law
The ratio between **increment threshold** and background **luminance** is limited by quantal fluctuations under **scotopic** viewing conditions. Threshold is proportional to the square root of background intensity. For **photopic** viewing conditions, **Weber's law** applies. *Synonym is **square root law**.*

decentration
Movement of a contact lens away from the centre of the **cornea**. With **rigid gas permeable** lenses, indicates a flat fit or an excessively thick lens.

decussation
Crossing over (of nerve fibres).

deep anterior lamellar keratoplasty
Alternative to **penetrating keratoplasty** for treating **keratoconus**. The **Descemet's membrane** and **corneal endothelium** from the host cornea are left in place, to reduce the chances of rejection. *Acronym is **DALK**.*

deep learning
Advanced form of **machine learning** that utilises **neural network**s to automatically recognise which features of a dataset are relevant to solving a problem. Used in image classification.

delayed optokinetic nystagmus
The portion of **optokinetic nystagmus** that gradually builds in velocity. This form of optokinetic nystagmus is responsible for **optokinetic after-nystagmus**. *Abbreviation is **OKNd**.*

dellen
Localised **corneal** thinning, usually near the **limbus**, caused by dehydration of the **corneal stroma**. *Synonym is **Fuchs' dimple**.*

Demer pulley
Theoretical pulleys which are supposedly involved in movement of the eye.

demodex
Tiny mites that can live in **eyelash** follicles and cause dry eye syndrome.

D

dendrite
Input branches of a neuron. From the Greek for 'root'.

dendropsia
Visual **hallucination** causing perception of branching patterns.

deorsumduction
Synonym of ***infraduction***.

depiction theory
Traditional theory that the visual system aims to provide a **veridical** representation of objective physical space. See also **interface theory**.

depression
Looking down.

depressor
A muscle that causes **depression** of the eye.

depth of field
The axial range over which the object plane can be moved without noticing image deterioration.

depth of focus
The axial range over which the image plane can be moved without noticing image deterioration.

dermatochalasis
Sagging of the skin of either **eyelid**, common with age. Can cause a visual obstruction if severe.

dermoid
A fleshy mass found on the **conjunctiva**. Smaller than **lipodermoid**.

Descemet's membrane
A structureless layer of the **cornea**; found between the **corneal endothelium** and **Dua's layer**. 6–12 μm thick.

Descemet's stripping endothelial keratoplasty
Transplant of just the **Descemet's membrane** and **corneal endothelium** – rejection less likely than in complete **keratoplasty**. *Acronym is DSEK.*

detection acuity
The ability to discern if a stimulus is present or not. *Synonym is* ***discrimination acuity.***

deturgescence
The relative dehydration of the **corneal stroma** that allows the **cornea** to maintain its transparent properties.

deutan
Refers to both **deuteranopes** and **deuteranomalopes**.

deuteranomalope
An individual with a **deuteranomaly**.

deuteranomaly
Anomalous trichromatism in which more green is required for colour matching. Common.

deuteranope
An individual with **deuteranopia**.

deuteranopia
Dichromatism in which there is no **chlorolabe** pigment.

dextrocycloversion
Rotating eye movement in which the upper **corneal** poles of both eyes rotate to the patient's right.

dextroversion
Movement of both eyes to the right.

DHD
Acronym of dissociated horizontal divergence.

diabetic maculopathy
Oedema and **exudates**. Causes **visual impairment**. Three types: **focal diabetic maculopathy, diffuse diabetic maculopathy**, and **ischaemic diabetic maculopathy**.

diabetic retinopathy
Retinal changes in response to diabetes mellitus. Severity is graded as **background diabetic retinopathy, pre-proliferative diabetic retinopathy**, and **proliferative diabetic retinopathy**. *Acronym is DR.*

diaphoresis
Excessive sweating.

dichoptic presentation
Presentation (of a visual stimulus) to both eyes simultaneously.

dichotomous test
Describes any test that puts people into two distinct groups.

dichromatism
Condition in which one type of photoreceptor is not present or does not work at all.

diclofenac
A **NSAID**.

diencephalon
At the midline of the brain, above the brainstem. Derived from the prosencephalon.

difference threshold
Synonym of ***increment threshold***.

diffractive contact lens
Type of **simultaneous vision contact lens** with structure on lens surface causing image diffraction into two powers which are perceived simultaneously.

diffractive intraocular lens
Uses interference patterns. Gives good near and good distance vision.

diffuse cerebral oedema
Swelling of the brain as a whole.

diffuse choroidal atrophy
Rare condition similar to **choroideraemia**.

diffuse diabetic maculopathy
Loss of **foveal** depression, thickened retina, multiple areas of **cystoid macular oedema** (cobblestone effect). *Synonym is* ***cystoid diabetic maculopathy***.

diffuse drusen
Synonym of ***soft drusen***.

diffuse episcleritis
Episcleritis that is not nodular. *Synonym is* ***simple episcleritis***.

diffuse lamellar keratitis
Complication of laser eye surgery in which sterile inflammation of the **corneal** wound occurs, usually a few days after surgery. Causes pain, reduced **visual acuity**, and a change in corneal topography with a hyperopic shift.

diffusion tensor imaging
Magnetic resonance imaging technique producing structural maps of white matter tractography. **Fractional anisotropy** of water molecules is measured at each voxel, and probable tracts are inferred from the data. *Acronym is* ***DTI***.

diktyoma
Synonym of ***medulloepithelioma***.

dilatation
Synonym of ***mydriasis***.

dilation
*Synonym of **mydriasis**.*

dilator pupillae
Thin layer of myoepithelium from the **iris root** to the **sphincter pupillae**. Contraction causes **mydriasis.**

dimple veil
Describes having several bubbles trapped under any type of contact lens; due to a bad fit.

dioptre
A measure of refractive power. Dioptric power is calculated by taking the inverse of the focal length of a lens, e.g. A lens with a focal length of 50 cm has a dioptric power of 1/0.5 = 2.00 D. *Abbreviation is **D**.*

dioptric telescope
*Synonym of **Galilean telescope**.*

diplopia
Double vision. *Adjective form is **diplopic**.*

diplopic
*Adjective form of **diplopia**.*

direct comparison eikenometer
A device that measures the extent of **aniseikonia.**

direct goniolens
Requires the patient to be **supine**. Abolishes the **critical angle** to provide direct view of **anterior chamber angle.**

direct tilt after-effect
Orientation-specific **receptive field**s can be fatigued, altering orientation perception. A **cortical** process.

disability glare
Glare that makes it very difficult to perform a task.

disc
*Synonym of **optic nerve head**.*

disc diameter
Unit of measurement used to indicate positions and sizes of **lesion**s on the **fundus**, using the **optic disc**'s size as a reference.

disc drusen
Calcium deposits under the **optic disc** (not the same kind of **drusen** as in **age-related macular degeneration**). *Synonym is **optic disc drusen**.*

disc haemorrhage
Synonym of ***splinter haemorrhage****.*

discomfort glare
Glare that does not cause inability to see but over time causes headaches, **photogenous asthenopia**, and other health problems.

discrimination acuity
Synonym of ***detection acuity****.*

disjunctive eye movement
Synonym of ***vergence****.*

dispenser's rule
When adjusting a patient's spectacles, for each degree of **pantoscopic tilt**, lower the ocular centre by 0.5 mm.

dissociated nystagmus
Nystagmus in which the oscillations of the eyes are of different amplitudes.

dissociated strabismus complex
Umbrella term for **dissociated vertical deviation**, dissociated horizontal deviation, and dissociated torsional deviation.

dissociated vertical deviation
A **dissociated strabismus complex** in which occluding either eye causes an elevated deviation. Occurs in **infantile esotropia syndrome**. *Acronym is* ***DVD****. Synonym is* ***alternating hyperphoria****.*

distance esotropia
Rare. Binocular single vision is present at near **fixation**, but there is an **esotropia** at distance.

distance exotropia
An intermittent **exotropia**: manifest in distance; binocular single vision at near. May be a **true distance exotropia** or a **simulated distance exotropia**.

distance Mallett unit
A **Mallett unit** for use at a viewing distance of six metres. *Acronym is* ***dMU****.*

distance penalisation
Over-plussing the better eye to encourage use of an eye with **amblyopia**.

distichiasis
A second row of **lash**es grow out of, or posterior to, the **meibomian gland** orifices.

divergence

The opposite of **convergence**. In reference to light: describes a **pencil** of rays that is becoming less focused. In relation to the eyes: describes a **vergence** eye movement in which the angle between the visual axes increases.

divergence fusional reserve

*Synonym of **negative fusional reserve**.*

Dk

Descriptor of the permeability of a material to gas. D = speed of gas diffusion, k = solubility of material to gas. Recorded in 'Fatt' units.

Dk/L

*Synonym of **Dk/t**.*

Dk/t

A contact lens's **Dk** divided by its total thickness (t, measured in cm). Dk/t is always reported for a –3.00 DS powered lens. *Synonym is **Dk/L**.*

DLEK

*Acronym of deep lamellar endothelial **keratoplasty**.*

DLK

*Acronym of deep lamellar **keratoplasty/diffuse lamellar keratitis**.*

DLPFC

*Acronym of **dorsolateral prefrontal cortex**.*

DLPN

Acronym of dorsolateral pontine nucleus.

DM

*Acronym of **diabetic maculopathy**/diabetes mellitus.*

DME

Acronym of diabetic macular oedema.

DMEK

*Acronym of **Descemet's membrane** endothelial keratoplasty.*

DMS

*Acronym of **dorsal midbrain syndrome**.*

dMU

*Acronym of **distance Mallett unit**.*

D

DO
Acronym of dispensing optician.

doll's eye reflex
Synonym of ***oculocephalic reflex****.*

dome magnifier
A type of **bright field magnifier**.

dominant drusen
Condition that presents in the 2nd–3rd decades of life. Causes yellow **drusen**. May cause **choroidal neovascularisation** and atrophy. *Synonyms are* ***Doyne's honeycomb dystrophy, familial dominant drusen,*** *and* ***malattia leventinese****.*

dominant optic atrophy
An autosomal dominantly inherited condition, first expressing between 6 and 12 years of age. Causes **disc** atrophy, colour vision loss, paracentral/**centrocaecal field defect**. *Synonyms are* ***autosomal dominant optic atrophy, juvenile optic atrophy,*** *and* ***Kjer's optic neuropathy****.*

Donders' classification
A series of classifications for **convergence/divergence** excess/insufficiencies.

Donders' strabismus
Synonym of ***fully accommodative esotropia****.*

Donders' law
Equal amounts of torsion occur no matter how an eye position is reached.

Donnan effect
Charged particles either side of a membrane will arrange to balance each other.

dorsal
Towards the back (of the body).

dorsal midbrain syndrome
Palsy of upgaze and **light-near dissociation**. Causes **convergence retraction saccadic pulses** and **Collier's sign**. Due to **lesion** of the **superior colliculus**, often by pineal tumour. *Acronym is DMS. Synonyms are* ***Parinaud-Koerber-Salus-Elschnig syndrome*** *and* ***Parinaud's syndrome****.*

dorsal stream
The 'where' pathway of visual processing. Incorporates **V3**, **visual area middle temporal**, **visual area medial superior temporal**, and the parietal cortex. *Synonym is* ***parietal stream****.*

dorsolateral prefrontal cortex
Brain area in the middle frontal gyrus involved in cognitive processes affecting eye movements, such as **saccadic inhibition** and anticipatory/predictive eye movements. *Acronym is DLPFC.*

dot haemorrhage
Haemorrhage in the **inner nuclear layer** of the retina.

double elevator palsy
Supranuclear **paresis** of **supraduction** (**superior rectus** and **inferior oblique**). **Bell's phenomenon** may be intact.

double Maddox rod test
A vertically oriented **Maddox rod** is placed in front of each eye (perceived as horizontal lines) – if vertical **diplopia** is present, one image will appear tilted; this can be used to diagnose the **paretic** muscle.

double opponent cells
Receptive fields which must be stimulated with more than one colour; e.g. R–G+ centre/ R+G– surround.

double saccadic pulse
A **saccadic pulse** in which the return to target is a **saccade**.

Doughty's classifications
Classifies artificial tears into 'simple' and 'complex', and eyewashes into 'emergency' and 'relief'.

Dowling–Rushton relationship
Log sensitivity during **dark adaptation** is linearly related to the concentration of bleached photopigment.

Down syndrome
Genetic disorder due to trisomy of chromosome 21. Causes characteristic facial appearance, with risk of high **ametropia** (usually **hyperopia**), inaccurate **accommodation, keratoconus, nystagmus**, and **strabismus**.

Doyne's honeycomb dystrophy
*Synonym of **dominant drusen**.*

DR
*Acronym of **diabetic retinopathy**.*

Drance haemorrhage
*Synonym of **splinter haemorrhage**.*

druse
*Singular of **drusen**.*

drusen
Extracellular material between **Bruch's membrane** and the **retinal pigment epithelium**. Reflection is caused by the thinner retina at the bulge. **AMD** is indicated by drusen >63 µm in conjunction with **RPE** changes. *Singular is **druse**.*

drusenoid pigment eipthelial detachment

A **pigment epithelium detachment** resulting from build-up of **drusen**.

dry age-related macular degeneration

The development of **drusen** at the **macula**r region. The drusen cause **metamorphopsia** and a gradual reduction in central **visual acuity**. Dry is the most common form of **age-related macular degeneration** and as yet is untreatable. May occur naturally in some individuals but is exacerbated by smoking, excessive sunlight exposure, and poor diet. *Synonyms are* ***atrophic age-related macular degeneration, geographic age-related macular degeneration****, and* ***non-exudative age-related macular degeneration****.*

DS

Acronym of dioptres of sphere.

DSAEK

Acronym of ***Descemet's stripping endothelial keratoplasty*** *(automated).*

DSE

Acronym of display screen equipment.

DSEK

Acronym of ***Descemet's stripping endothelial keratoplasty****.*

DTI

Acronym of ***diffusion tensor imaging****.*

DTL

Acronym of ***Dawson, Trick, Litzkow electrode****.*

Dua's layer

Layer of the **cornea** located between the **corneal stroma** and **Descemet's membrane**. Approximately 15 μm thick and acellular.

dual response theory

Rivalry and **fusion** are the same process; if fusion fails, switches to rivalry.

Duane's retraction syndrome

Congenital condition present in 1% of strabismics. Attempted **adduction** causes retraction of the **globe** and narrowing of **palpebral fissure**, due to neural miswiring. Considered both a mechanical and neurogenic restriction. Classified as any of **Duane's retraction syndrome type I, Duane's retraction syndrome type II, Duane's retraction syndrome type III**, or **Duane's retraction syndrome type C**. *Synonym is* ***Stilling–Türk syndrome****.*

Duane's retraction syndrome type A

Synonym of ***Duane's retraction syndrome type III****.*

Duane's retraction syndrome type B

Synonym of ***Duane's retraction syndrome type I****.*

Duane's retraction syndrome type C
Duane's retraction syndrome causing limited **adduction** and **abduction** to a lesser degree. Rare.

Duane's retraction syndrome type I
Duane's retraction syndrome causing limited **abduction**. Common. *Synonym is **Duane's retraction syndrome type B**.*

Duane's retraction syndrome type II
Duane's retraction syndrome causing limited **adduction.** Rare.

Duane's retraction syndrome type III
Duane's retraction syndrome causing limited **abduction** and **adduction** to a lesser degree. Common. *Synonym is **Duane's retraction syndrome type A**.*

duction
Movement of one eye.

dura mater
The outermost **meninx**, composed of durable connective tissue. At the optic nerve, has circular fibres in the centre, and longitudinal fibres on the outside.

DV
Acronym of distance vision.

DVD
*Acronym of **dissociated vertical deviation**.*

Dx
Abbreviation of diagnosis.

dye disappearance test
*Synonym of **Jones test**.*

dynamic contour tonometry
Tonometry in which the applanating surface matches the curvature of the **cornea**.

dynamic retinoscopy
Retinoscopy with a near **fixation** target. No working distance lens is required. A 'with' movement indicates an **accommodative lag**, whilst an 'against' movement indicates **accommodative lead**. There are two types: **Nott retinoscopy** and **monocular estimation method**.

dynamic visual acuity
Visual acuity for objects moving around the observer – often better than normal visual acuity, as processes can be sub**cortical**.

D

dysarthria
Inability to speak properly due to muscular problems.

dyschromatopsia
Any physical impairment of colour vision, such as **dichromatism**, **anomalous trichromatism**, or **achromatopsia**. *Synonym is **colour deficiency**.*

dyscrasia
From the Greek for 'bad mix': refers to any blood disorder.

dysfibrinogenemia
Dysfunctional **fibrinogen**.

dysgenesis
*Synonym of **hypoplasia**.*

dysgraphia
Inability to write, despite having the intellectual ability and knowledge. Linked to dyslexia. *Synonym is **agraphia**.*

dysmegalopsia
*Synonym of **dysmetropsia**.*

dysmetric saccade
Hypometric saccades and/or **hypermetric saccades**.

dysmetropsia
Perceptual spatial distortion including **macropsia**, **micropsia**, **pelopsia**, and **teleopsia**. *Synonym is **dysmegalopsia**.*

dysphasia
Impaired speech and comprehension of speech.

dysplasia
Change in size, shape, and organisation of the cells of a tissue.

dysthyroid optic neuropathy
Optic nerve damage resulting from **thyroid eye disease**.

dystrophia epithelialis corneae
Corneal stromal oedema seen in advanced **Fuchs' endothelial dystrophy**.

E

E
*Abbreviation of energy/**esophoria/illuminance**.*

E(T)
*Abbreviation of intermittent **esotropia**.*

early onset macular dystrophy
*Synonym of **Leber's congenital amaurosis**.*

early optokinetic nystagmus
The portion of **optokinetic nystagmus** that responds immediately to a large moving stimulus. *Abbreviation is **OKNe**.*

early receptor potential
A fluctuation seen in electroretinography, due to photoisomerisation of photopigment. Only seen when patient is dark-adapted. Biphasic. *Acronym is **ERP**.*

easy V
*Synonym of **mini bevel**.*

eccentric fixation
The use of an area of the retina other than **foveola** to view straight-ahead (even **monocular**ly). *Acronym is EF.*

eccentric viewing
The practice of actively looking to the side of something to view it, usually due to **foveal** damage. Individuals are aware they are doing this, as opposed to **eccentric fixation**. *Acronym is EV.*

echography
Ultrasound used to investigate axial length, **pachymetry**, and to scan for **intraocular** tumour/foreign body. *Synonym is **ultrasound scan**.*

eclampsia
Pre-eclampsia when it occurs in conjunction with seizures.

eclipse technique
A pen torch is shone at 90° from the eye; the shadow of the iris on the other side is used to estimate **anterior chamber angle** (graded from IV to I).

ECT
Acronym of electroconvulsive therapy.

ectasia
Synonym of ***corneal ectasia****.*

ectoparasite
A parasite that lives on an organism.

ectopia lentis
Synonym of ***ectopia lentis et pupillae****.*

ectopia lentis et pupillae
Any **luxation** or **subluxation** of the lens. *Synonym is* ***ectopia lentis****.*

ectopic macula
Displaced **macula**. Can lead to reduced **visual acuity**, **metamorphopsia**, or **strabismus**.

ectopic pupil
Synonym of ***corectopia****.*

ectropion
An out-turned lower **eyelid**.

ectropion uveae
Iris turns out; posterior iris is drawn round **pupillary margin** to anterior iris. Can occur in **neurofibromatosis type 1**.

Edinger–Westphal/oculomotor pupil
No **pupil** reflex at all. The involved pupil is usually larger.

Edinger–Westphal nucleus
Nucleus of the parasympathetic division of the **oculomotor nerve** (leading to **ciliary ganglion**).

Edridge-Green lantern
A **lantern test** that is no longer used.

EDTA
Acronym of ***ethylene diamine tetraacetic acid****.*

EE
Acronym of eye examination.

EF
Acronym of ***eccentric fixation****.*

effectivity
The fact that **vergence** changes throughout a **pencil**.

efference copy
The expected result of motor innervation, e.g. movement of the world following a signal for the eyes to move. *Synonym is **corollary discharge.***

efferent nerve
A nerve that carries a signal away from the central nervous system. *Opposite of **afferent nerve.***

Egger's line
The line formed by **Wieger's ligament**.

egocentric subjective visual direction
*Synonym of **absolute subjective visual direction.***

egocentric unilateral neglect
Unilateral neglect of all of the visual scene in one half of the **visual field**.

Ehler's formula
Used to relate **central corneal thickness** to **intraocular pressure**.

Ehlers–Danlos syndrome
Collagen abnormality causing hypermobile joints. Causes **myopia** and **ectopia lentis**. Associated with **keratoconus**.

eigengrau
*Synonym of **intrinsic light.***

eigenlicht
*Synonym of **intrinsic light.***

EK
*Acronym of endothelial **keratoplasty.***

EKC
*Acronym of **epidemic keratoconjunctivitis.***

electro-oculogram dark trough
Minimum standing potential of the eye found when dark-adapted for ~12 mins.

electro-oculogram light peak
Maximum standing potential of the eye found after 8–12 mins in the light.

electro-oculography
Technique that measures the **corneoretinal potential**. Assesses the **retinal pigment epithelium** and photoreceptors. The patient is made to look left and right during the procedure. Can also be used as an **eye tracking** technique. *Acronym is **EOG.***

E

electroretinography
Technique that measures electrical signals evoked from various parts of the retina. *Acronym is ERG.*

elevation
Looking up.

elevator
1. Height adjustment that is applied to a **visual field** plot to calculate the **pattern deviation map**. It is the 7th value from the list of ranked values.
2. A muscle that causes **elevation** of the eye.

Elschnig pearl
Type of **posterior capsular opacification** caused by **proliferation** of the remaining epithelial cells over the **lens capsule** following **cataract** surgery.

Elschnig spots
Small yellowish spots found on the **fundus** in **hypertensive choroidopathy** due to **choroid**al **ischaemia**.

Elschnig's rim
The area around the **optic nerve head** that is slightly paler than the retina, sometimes mistaken for part of the optic nerve head.

embolism
The blockage of a vessel with something that has been carried around the bloodstream, e.g. blood clot.

embolus
An abnormal object that travels around the bloodstream that has the potential to block blood vessels (causing an **embolism**).

embryogenesis
The process by which the embryo as a whole develops.

embryonic induction
A part of the embryo sending a signal to another part to induce development of that part.

emission theory
The rebutted theory that visual perception is achieved by emission of light from the eyes. *Synonym is **extramission theory**.*

emmetropia
The case in which there is no refractive error in the eye with **accommodation** relaxed, and parallel light is focused at the retina.

emmetropisation
The natural process of human development that causes children to change from **hyperopia** to almost **emmetropia** in the first few years of life.

empirical horopter
*Synonym of **subjective fronto-parallel plane**.*

enantiomorphism
Mirror image symmetry.

encephalotrigeminal angiomatosis
*Synonym of **Sturge–Weber syndrome**.*

end-point nystagmus
Physiological **nystagmus** in which a slow drift away from the point of **fixation** followed by a quick-phase refixation occurs when attempting to look in extremes of **gaze**. Believed to be due to a leaky **neural integrator** (low gain). Increases in amplitude with alcohol intoxication.

end-stopped cell
Type of cell found in the **primary visual cortex** and **extrastriate cortex** with **receptive fields** that detect motion of oriented edges of specific lengths (useful in detecting moving corners). *Synonym is **hypercomplex cell**.*

endocrine signalling
Cellular messaging system which utilises hormones.

endomysium
A layer of connective tissue that surrounds individual muscle fibres.

endoparasite
A parasite that lives inside an organism.

endophthalmitis
Inflammation of the inside of the eye. An unfortunate complication of **intraocular** surgery, usually occurring after 3 days.

endophthalmos
*Synonym of **enophthalmos**.*

endophytic
Growing inwards.

endosteum
Lines the inner cavity of bones.

endotoxins
Formed by dead bacteria cell walls. Can cause disease.

enhanced monovision
Having a bifocal or **multifocal contact lens** in one eye and a single vision contact lens in the fellow eye.

enhanced readers
A regressive lens with the reading **addition** at the bottom and an intermediate reading addition at the top of the lens.

enhanced trabeculectomy
The **trabeculectomy** bleb is cured with a chemical to prevent healing (i.e. scarring over).

enophthalmos
Recession of the **globe** into the **orbit**. Can occur with a **blowout fracture** or as a result of **oculo-digital sign**. *Synonym is **endophthalmos**.*

ENT
Acronym of ear, nose, and throat.

entoptic phenomena
*Plural of **entoptic phenomenon**.*

entoptic phenomenon
Any visual phenomena whose origin is within the eye, e.g. **floaters**, **Haidinger's brush**, the **blue field entoptic phenomenon**, **phosphene**s, **Maxwell's spot**, **Purkinje blue arcs**, and the **Purkinje tree**. *Plural is **entoptic phenomena**.*

entoptoscope
A bright light source viewed through a small aperture. Allows the observer to experience **entoptic phenomena** more easily.

entropion
An in-turned lower **eyelid**.

enucleation
Removal of the eye, usually leaving the **extraocular muscle**s and the other **orbit**al contents.

EOG
*Acronym of **electro-oculography**.*

EOM
*Acronym of **extraocular muscle**.*

EOP
*Acronym of **equivalent oxygen pressure**.*

epi-LASIK
The **microkeratome** only cuts into the **corneal epithelium**, separating it from the **corneal stroma**.

epi-off

Corneal cross-linking in which the **corneal epithelium** is removed.

epi-on

Corneal cross-linking in which the **corneal epithelium** is not removed.

epiblast

Cells formed near the trophoblasts after embryonic invasion of the uterus wall.

epiblepharon

Extra fold of skin in the lower **eyelid**. Can (rarely) cause **trichiasis**. Often resolves as patient grows.

epicanthal fold

Skin fold in the upper **eyelid** present in Asian individuals and all human foetuses. Reduction of its prominence is due to growth of the nose.

epicanthus inversus

Case in which the lower **palpebral furrow** is more prominent than the upper palpebral furrow.

epicapsular star

Small brown star-shaped deposits on lens. Not a problem unless there are so many that **visual acuity** is compromised.

epidemic keratoconjunctivitis

Highly contagious **inflammation** of both the **cornea** and **conjunctiva** due to **adenovirus** infection. *Acronym is EKC.*

epilation

Hair removal (can refer to **eyelash** removal).

epimysium

Layer of tissue that covers the whole of a skeletal muscle.

epiphora

Spillage of tears onto the cheeks. Either due to excessive lacrimation or insufficient tear drainage. Often due to blocked **nasolacrimal duct**.

epiphysis

The joining end of a long bone.

epiretinal membrane

The formation of scar tissue at the **macula** which can stretch, causing **metamorphopsia** and a slight decrease in **visual acuity**. In a mild form, it is known as 'cellophane maculopathy', and in a severe form, it is known as 'macular pucker'. *Synonyms are **idiopathic premacular fibrosis** and **preretinal membrane**.*

episclera
The outermost layer of the **sclera**, made of loose connective tissue and small blood vessels.

episcleritis
Causes redness and discomfort. Frequently recurring benign condition, most common in women between 20 and 40 years of age. If particularly uncomfortable, anti-inflammatories are sometimes prescribed. It is very important to differentiate the condition from the much more serious **scleritis**.

epithelial basement membrane dystrophy
Synonym of ***Cogan's microcystic dystrophy.***

epithelial microcysts
Indicator of chronic **corneal hypoxia**. Seen as grey dots on the **corneal epithelium**. Often due to contact lens wear.

epoxy resin
A glass cement sometimes used in spectacles.

equidistance tendency
Phenomenon describing the fact that observers tend to perceive objects in adjacent parts of the **visual field** as being at a similar distance to one another. Partially explains the **moon illusion**.

equitint
A layer of tint which is applied on one surface of an ophthalmic lens to provide even coverage.

equivalent background theory
During **dark adaptation**, sensitivity is equal to that caused by **adaptation** to a background light.

equivalent oxygen percentage
Synonym of ***equivalent oxygen pressure.***

equivalent oxygen pressure
The concentration of oxygen that induces an equivalent oxygen 'thirst' of the **cornea**. *Acronym is* ***EOP****. Synonym is* ***equivalent oxygen percentage.***

equivalent sphere
Half of an ophthalmic cylinder's power. Indicates the midpoint of the astigmatic **pencil** produced by the cylindrical portion of a lens.

ERG
Acronym of ***electroretinography.***

ERP
Acronym of ***early receptor potential.***

erythrolabe
The photosensitive pigment present in **L-cones**.

erythropsia
Red **chromatopsia**.

eso
Refers to either **esophoria** or **esotropia**.

esophoria
Horizontal **heterophoria** in which the eyes have a latent inward turn.

esotropia
Horizontal **strabismus** in which the non-fixating eye is turned inward. *Abbreviation is **ET**.*

essential anisocoria
Insignificant **anisocoria**. 20% of people have some level of anisocoria, usually less than 1 mm. The cause is unknown.

essential hypertension
Hypertension with no known cause (90–95% of all hypertensive patients). *Synonym is **primary hypertension**.*

ester-linked anaesthetic
Degraded faster than **amide-linked anaesthetics** because esterases are present in the eye. Lasts ~20–30 mins in the eye. Examples include **proxymetacaine, oxybuprocaine**, and **tetracaine**.

Esterman test
Perimetry test done at a fixed brightness of 10 dB across the whole retina.

ET
*Abbreviation of **esotropia**.*

ETDRS
Acronym of the early treatment of diabetic retinopathy study.

ethmoid bone
Small bone that separates the nasal cavity from the brain. Located between the **orbits**.

ethmoid sinuses
Between the nose and eyes, in the **ethmoid bone**. One of the paranasal **sinuses**.

ethylene diamine tetraacetic acid
Preservative found in some contact lens solutions; its main purpose is to chelate calcium and magnesium. *Acronym is **EDTA**.*

etiology
The study of causation.

euthyroidism
Normal functioning of thyroid gland. ~10% of patients with mild **thyroid eye disease** are euthyroid.

EV
Acronym of ***eccentric viewing****.*

evaporimetry
A non-clinical tear film test; measures how fast the tear film evaporates.

EVES
Acronym of electronic vision enhancement system.

evisceration
Removal of the internal organs. In reference to the eyes, removal of the ocular contents, retaining the **sclera** and **extraocular muscle**s.

EW
Acronym of ***Edinger–Westphal nucleus****/extended wear.*

excimer laser
Ultraviolet laser that neither burns nor cuts – just disrupts molecular bonds; 'cold laser'.

exclusive dominance
The case in binocular vision in which one (small) stimulus is ignored completely in favour of another.

excycloduction
Monocular **extorsion**.

excyclophoria
Latent deviation in which the top of the eye drifts in a temporal direction.

excyclorotation
Synonym of ***extorsion****.*

excyclotropia
Manifest deviation in which the top of the eye drifts in a temporal direction.

excyclovergence
Eye movement in which the upper **corneal** poles of both eyes rotate outward.

exenteration
Enucleation and removal of the orbital contents.

exfoliation syndrome
Synonym of ***pseudoexfoliation syndrome.***

exit pupil
Virtual point in an optical system from which all light emerges.

exo
Refers to either **exophoria** or **exotropia**.

exophoria
Horizontal **heterophoria** in which the eyes have a latent outward turn. *Abbreviation is X.*

exophthalmos
Synonym of ***proptosis.***

exophytic
Growing outwards.

exotropia
Horizontal **strabismus** in which the non-fixating eye is turned outward. *Abbreviation is XT.*

expansion prism
A prismatic lens addition designed for patients with **homonymous hemianopia** to help them retrieve lost **visual field** by directing their **gaze** towards the prism. Two designs exist: the **Peli lens** and the **Gottlieb visual field awareness system**.

express saccade
A **saccade** with extremely fast reaction time – usually in response to a new stimulus presented following a short gap in which no stimulus is visible.

exproprioception
Information gained through both **proprioception** and **exteroception**, i.e. the position of the body in relation to the world.

expulsive haemorrhage
Rare complication of **cataract** extraction in which **intraocular pressure** increases, and contents of eye haemorrhage through the incision.

extended duration plug
A synthetic temporary **punctal** plug. Lasts ~10–12 weeks.

extended reality
Umbrella term for both **augmented reality** and **virtual reality**. *Acronym is XR.*

external hordeolum
A **hordeolum** affecting a lash follicle and **Zeis glands** or **Moll glands**. *Synonym is stye.*

E

external limiting membrane
*Synonym of **outer limiting membrane**.*

exteroception
Information about the layout of an environment.

extorsion
Eye rotation temporally. If constantly present, may be caused by weakness of the **superior oblique**. *Synonym is **excyclorotation**. Verb form is **extort**.*

extort
*Verb form of **extorsion**.*

extrafusal muscle fibres
The fibres of skeletal muscles. Innervated by alpha-motor neurons.

extrageniculostriate cortex
*Synonym of **retinotectal pathway**.*

extramission theory
*Synonym of **emission theory**.*

extraocular muscle
Any of the six muscles that control the movement of each eye: the **medial rectus**, **lateral rectus**, **superior rectus**, **inferior rectus**, **superior oblique**, and **inferior oblique**. *Acronym is EOM.*

extrastriate body area
Region of the **extrastriate cortex** that encodes for visual recognition of body parts.

extrastriate cortex
The **visual cortex** except for the **primary visual cortex**, comprising Brodmann areas 18 and 19, which defines the areas **V2**, **V3**, **V4**, and **V5**. *Synonyms are **visual association area** and **visual association cortex**.*

exudate
A liquid or semisolid discharged to a surface or into a cavity.

exudation
Slow oozing of a liquid from a vessel.

exudative age-related macular degeneration
*Synonym of **wet age-related macular degeneration**.*

exudative diabetic maculopathy
*Synonym of **focal diabetic maculopathy**.*

exudative retinal detachment
*Synonym of **serous retinal detachment**.*

eye tracker
Device used for **eye tracking.** Most modern systems are video-based and involve tracking the pupil and corneal reflection; other techniques include **electro-oculography** and the **scleral search coil**.

eye tracking
Measurement of gaze direction or eye movement over time, by an **eye tracker**.

eyeball
*Synonym of **globe**.*

eyelash
*Synonym of **cilium**.*

eyelashes
*Synonym of **cilia**.*

eyelid
Either one of the protective sheets that moves over the surface of the eye to restore the tear film, to protect the eye from damage, and to drain tears from the surface of the eye. *Plural is **blephara**. Synonyms are **blepharon** and **palpebra**.*

F

F
Abbreviation of ***luminous flux****/dioptric power.*

F–M 100
Acronym of ***Farnsworth–Munsell 100 hue test****.*

FA
Acronym of ***fractional anisotropy****.*

facial nerve
Cranial nerve VII. Paralysis of this nerve is known as **Bell's palsy**. *Synonym is* ***seventh cranial nerve****.*

facial sheath of the eye
Synonym of ***Tenon's capsule****.*

facility of accommodation
Synonym of ***accommodative facility****.*

FALANT test
Synonym of ***Farnsworth lantern test****.*

false alarm
In **signal detection theory**, the situation in which a response is generated by a noise stimulus, i.e. a **hallucination**.

false negative response
In **perimetry**, no response to a high luminance stimulus where higher sensitivity was found earlier in the test.

false positive response
In **perimetry**, response to a non-stimulus or a response faster than patient's normal response speed.

familial dominant drusen
Synonym of ***dominant drusen****.*

far distance
Describes a test done in which 'distance' is more than 6 metres away – may be relevant with some forms of **strabismus**.

far field diffraction
Synonym of ***Fraunhofer diffraction****.*

farinata
Synonym of ***corneal farinata.***

Farnsworth D15 test
A colour vision test with 15 caps to be arranged in order of hue. Good for detecting **tritans**.

Farnsworth lantern test
A **lantern test**, most commonly used in aviation. *Synonym is* ***FALANT test.***

Farnsworth–Munsell 100 hue test
A colour vision test similar to the **Farnsworth D15 test** but involving 85 coloured discs, for greater accuracy. Also known as '100 hue test', despite only having 85 discs. *Acronym is* ***F–M 100.***

farsightedness
Synonym of ***hyperopia.***

fascia
Type of connective tissue that surrounds and gives support to muscles.

fascia bulbi
Synonym of ***Tenon's capsule.***

fascicle
A bundle of skeletal muscle fibres.

fast fusion
Binocular **fusion** that overcomes **diplopia** in approximately one second but cannot be maintained. Caused by **retinal slip**.

FASTPAC
An algorithm for the **Humphrey field analyser** which decreases stimulus by 3 dB until seen.

fatigue effect
Over time, patients will do worse in **perimetry** if they have a moderate defect, and marginally worse in normal areas and the periphery, due to fatigue.

Fatt method
Synonym of ***polarographic method.***

Fatt units
The units in which Dk (permeability of a contact lens material to gas) is measured. *Synonym is* ***Barrer units.***

FAZ
Acronym of foveal avascular zone.

FB
Acronym of foreign body.

FD
Acronym of ***fixation disparity.***

FDDT
Acronym of ***fluorescein dye disappearance test.***

FDT
Acronym of ***frequency doubling technology.***

feature analysis theory
Theory of perception stating that we recognise objects by analysing the features and combining them.

Fechner's law
Perceived stimulus intensity is proportional to the logarithm of stimulus intensity.

feeler
Piece of copper wire used to lower the **button** into the **contact curve** in a fused bifocal.

FEF
Acronym of ***frontal eye fields.***

femtosecond LASIK
Stromal flap is created with a femtosecond laser (not a **microkeratome**). Similar patient selection criteria to LASIK.

Ferry–Porter law
Critical flicker fusion frequency increases linearly with the log of the stimulus luminance.

FFA
Acronym of ***fundus fluorescein angiography.***

FH
Acronym of family history.

FHC
Acronym of ***Fuchs' heterochromia cyclitis.***

fibrillogenesis
Development of the fibrils present in collagen.

fibrinogen
Produces fibrin, which clots blood.

fibrinolysis
Removal of fibrin and **fibrinogen** by plasmin.

fibrinoplatelet emboli
Multiple grey particles; sometimes fill vessel lumen. Sometimes permanent. Can cause **amaurosis fugax**.

fibroblast
Maintain structural integrity of connective tissue by continually secreting extracellular matrix.

fibronectin
Glycoprotein that binds to **integrins**.

fibrosis
Development of excess fibrous connective tissue.

field of binocular single vision
The extent to which a person can **gaze** whilst maintaining binocular single vision.

fifth cranial nerve
Synonym of ***trigeminal nerve***.

figure-ground segmentation
The way in which objects stand out from each other due to differences in colour and **contrast**.

filamentary keratitis
Keratitis in which **corneal epithelium** filaments pass into the **corneal stroma**. Most fungal infections show this.

Filehne effect
Perceived movement of the background when tracking a moving object.

filtering operation
Synonym of ***trabeculectomy***.

filtration surgery
Synonym of ***trabeculectomy***.

Fincham–Sutcliffe screener
A type of wall-mounted multiple stimulus **perimeter**.

fingerprint dystrophy
Synonym of ***Cogan's microcystic dystrophy***.

FIPTs
Acronym of ***focal intraretinal periarteriolar transudates***.

F

first focal length
Distance from a positive lens at which the **focal point** lies (when incident light is parallel).

Fisher syndrome
*Synonym of **Miller Fisher syndrome**.*

fixation
Maintaining **gaze** on a fixed **location** in physical space.

fixation disparity
Condition in which the two eyes don't fixate with corresponding parts of the retina; images may be seen as double if the points don't lie within **Panum's fusional area**. Many individuals have a small degree of fixation disparity. *Acronym is **FD**. Synonym is **retinal disparity**.*

fixed doubling keratometer
*Synonym of **two position keratometer**.*

flame haemorrhage
Haemorrhage in the **nerve fibre layer**. Found in **hypertensive retinopathy**.

flash coating
Method of tinting high index lenses (only CR39 can be dyed) – metal spattered on.

flash electroretinogram
Electroretinography using a flashed stimulus – primarily assesses the peripheral retina.

flash-induced nystagmus
Nystagmus induced by viewing high frequency monocular flashes of light. The nystagmus beats in the direction of the stimulated eye.

flash visual evoked potential
Most complex type of **visual evoked potential**. Contains four negative peaks and two positive.

flat field magnifier
*Synonym of **bright field magnifier**.*

Fleischer ring
Pigmented ring visible on the **cornea**, indicative of **keratoconus**.

Flexner–Wintersteiner rosettes
Histological appearance of **retinoblastoma** tumour cells.

flicker fusion test
*Synonym of **critical flicker fusion frequency**.*

flip-up spectacles
Spectacles with a reading **addition** attached in a flip-down device.

floaters
Entoptic phenomenon caused by debris floating around the **vitreous humour**. Perception of these is called **myodesopsia**.

flocculus
Part of the cerebellum, receives signals from the middle ear and regulates balance and eye movement.

floppy eyelid syndrome
Occurs most often in obese elderly males. **Eyelid** is so loose it can be everted in sleep; painful.

fluorescein
Synonym of ***sodium fluorescein***.

fluorescein angiography
Sodium fluorescein is injected into the bloodstream, a cobalt blue filter is used in conjunction with a **fundus** camera to take timed photographs which can show leakage from vessels in the eye. *Synonym is* ***fundus fluorescein angiography***.

fluorescein break-up time test
The external eye is treated with **sodium fluorescein**; the time taken for the tears to visibly break-up is noted. <5 seconds indicates dry eye, <10 seconds is borderline.

fluorescein dye disappearance test
Synonym of ***Jones test***.

fluoret
A paper strip impregnated with **sodium fluorescein**.

fluorexon
A stain similar to **sodium fluorescein** which is less readily taken up by soft contact lenses as it has a larger molecular size. Unfortunately it does not stain as well.

flying corpuscle test
The blue light of an entoptoscope is shone at the patient. Normal **macular** function is diagnosed if at least 15 white blood cells are perceived by the patient.

Flynn phenomenon
Constriction of the pupil in response to darkness. Sometimes seen in retinal disorders such as **Leber's congenital amaurosis** and **achromatopsia**.

flyover vessel
A vessel that no longer lies in contact with the retina at the cup due to cup nerve cell loss.

FMNS
*Acronym of **fusion maldevelopment nystagmus syndrome**.*

fMRI
*Acronym of **functional magnetic resonance imaging**.*

focal adhesion
Protein complexes that bind cells to the extracellular matrix. Utilises **integrins**.

F

focal diabetic maculopathy
More common in type 2 diabetes. Circumscribed retinal thickening and circinate **hard exudates**. *Synonym is **exudative diabetic maculopathy**.*

focal intraretinal periarteriolar transudates
Punctate white opacities found alongside arterioles. Due to malignant **hypertension**. *Acronym is **FIPTs**.*

focal length
The distance from a lens at which parallel light is focused.

focal point
The exact point in physical space at which a **pencil** of rays is perfectly in focus.

focus of expansion
The origin of **optic flow**. *Acronym is **FoE**.*

FoE
*Acronym of **focus of expansion**.*

FOH
Acronym of family ocular history.

follicles
Nodular swellings of the **tarsal conjunctiva** without a vascular tuft due to white blood cell build-up (viral infection).

follicular conjunctivitis
Usually unilateral; **follicles** on **conjunctiva**.

foramen
An opening through a bone.

foramen magnum
Hole in the occipital bones where the medulla oblongata enters from the spine.

forced duction test
The **conjunctiva** is physically grabbed and moved to see if a restriction of movement is mechanical or neurological in origin.

form fit plug
*Synonym of **smart plug**.*

fornix
Join between the **bulbar conjunctiva** and **palpebral conjunctiva**.

fornix conjunctiva
The part of the **conjunctiva** covering the **fornix**.

Forsius–Eriksson syndrome
*Synonym of **Åland Island disease**.*

Forster–Fuchs' spot
*Synonym of **Fuchs' spot**.*

fortification spectra
*Synonym of **teichopsia**.*

fossa
A broad, shallow, depressed area in bone.

Fourier analysis
Breakdown of a stimulus into sine waves for each **spatial frequency**.

Fourier domain optical coherence tomography
*Synonym of **spectral domain optical coherence tomography**.*

Fourier synthesis
Recombination of different **spatial frequency** pathways into a single image (in the brain).

fourth cranial nerve
*Synonym of **trochlear nerve**.*

FoV
*Acronym of **field of view**.*

fovea
Depression at the centre of the **macula** at which, in normals, **visual acuity** is highest. *Synonym is **fovea centralis**.*

fovea centralis
*Synonym of **fovea**.*

F

fovea plana
Absence of the **foveal** pit. Often occurs in conjunction with visual impairment but can be present in individuals with good **visual acuity**. *Synonym is* ***foveal hypoplasia***.

foveal hypoplasia
Synonym of ***fovea plana***.

foveola
Central part of **fovea** that is exclusively cone-dominated.

FOZD
Acronym of front optic zone diameter.

FOZR
Acronym of front optic zone radius.

FPR
Acronym of front peripheral radius.

FR
Acronym of ***fusional reserve***.

fractional anisotropy
Measure of the direction of diffusion of a molecule. 0 = equal diffusion in all directions; 1 = diffusion only in one direction. Used in **diffusion tensor imaging** as a measure of water diffusion. *Acronym is* ***FA***.

frame of reference
Enough information to facilitate binocular vision between two images.

Franceschetti's oculo-digital sign
Synonym of ***oculo-digital sign***.

Fraunhofer diffraction
Diffraction patterns occurring in the image plane (in focus). *Synonym is* ***far field diffraction***.

Freeman plug
An extracanalicular **puncta**l plug.

Frenzel spectacles
Spectacles containing high positive lenses and lights between the lenses and the eyes, used for the close inspection of **nystagmus**. They also prevent gaze fixation which may suppress some forms of nystagmus.

frequency domain optical coherence tomography
Optical coherence tomography calculated using **Fourier analysis**; no need to move reference mirror, faster, and gives 3D image.

frequency doubling technology
An alternating sine wave grating is used to measure **visual fields**. Primarily measures the response of magno-gamma cells, which are supposedly affected early in **glaucoma**. *Acronym is FDT.*

Fresnel diffraction
Diffraction patterns anywhere except at the in-focus plane.

Fresnel lens
Poor quality image but a huge magnification without a bulky lens. Used in lighthouses. *Synonym is* ***Fresnel prism.***

Fresnel prism
Synonym of ***Fresnel lens.***

Frisby test
Stereopsis test that uses physically different depths to assess stereopsis.

frontal bone
The forehead and top part of the **orbit**.

frontal eye fields
One of the **cortical eye fields**. Receives input from **visual area medial superior temporal**, parietal cortex, **supplemental eye fields**, and **lateral intraparietal area**. Contains two subregions: the **superior frontal eye fields** and **inferior frontal eye fields**. *Acronym is FEF.*

frontal plane
Synonym of ***coronal plane.***

frontal sinuses
Above the eyes. One of the paranasal **sinus**es.

frontalis muscle
Starts at the top of the head. Attaches to and moves eyebrow.

FS
Acronym of foveal suppression.

FSP
Acronym of front surface power.

FTMH
Acronym of ***full-thickness macular hole.***

Fuchs' crypts
Depressions near the **collarette** of the iris.

F

Fuchs' dimple
*Synonym of **dellen**.*

Fuchs' dystrophy
*Synonym of **Fuchs' endothelial dystrophy**.*

Fuchs' endothelial dystrophy
Bilateral dystrophy of **Descemet's membrane** and the **corneal endothelium**. Onset old age. **Guttata** and (eventually) **bullous keratopathy**. Vision worse in mornings. *Synonym is **Fuchs' dystrophy**.*

Fuchs' heterochromia cyclitis
Iridocyclitis leading to **heterochromia** due to iris atrophy. May cause a secondary **glaucoma**. *Acronym is **FHC**.*

Fuchs' spot
Pigmented spot near the **macula** due to **choroidal neovascularisation** through **lacquer cracks**. *Synonym is **Forster–Fuchs' spot**.*

full threshold perimetry
Algorithm for the **Humphrey field analyser**; intensity goes down by 4 dB until seen, then up by 2 dB until not seen.

full-thickness macular hole
A macular hole spanning the entire retinal thickness from the **ILM** to the **RPE**. Most are **idiopathic full-thickness macular hole**s but may also be caused by myopia, trauma, or secondary to other disease/**iatrogenic** causes. *Acronym is **FTMH**.*

fully accommodative esotropia
Type of intermittent **esotropia**: esotropia when uncorrected, but with spectacles, binocular single vision at all distances. *Synonym is **Donders' strabismus**.*

functionaesa
Loss of function.

functional magnetic resonance imaging
Magnetic resonance imaging technique that measures changes in blood supply to active areas of brain to form a functional image of the brain. *Acronym is **fMRI**.*

fundus
The inner surface of the posterior eye, as viewed by **ophthalmoscopy**. Includes the retina and **optic nerve head**.

fundus albipunctatus
A possible cause of **congenital stationary nightblindness type II**. Flecky appearance to **fundus**. **Dark adaptation** takes a long time.

fundus flavimaculatus
Stargardt disease when it presents in the 4th–5th decades of life. Less severe but flecks throughout **fundus**.

fundus fluorescein angiography
Synonym of ***fluorescein angiography.***

fundus tigre
Synonym of ***tesselated fundus.***

funduscope
Synonym of ***ophthalmoscope.***

funduscopy
Synonym of ***ophthalmoscopy.***

fungal keratitis
Greyish-white, rough ulcers with feathery edges. Usually **filamentary keratitis** as well.

furrow degeneration
Asymptomatic degeneration causing peripheral **corneal ectasia**.

fused vergence fixation disparity curve
Plots **fixation disparity** against **associated phoria**; used to calculate prism or **spherical manipulation** to prescribe. *Acronym is* ***FVFDC.***

fusidic acid
An antibacterial, routinely used by **optometrist**s. Most effective against **Gram-positive** bacterium.

fusiform face area
Area of the brain where face recognition takes place.

fusion
Superimposition of (at least part of) the images from each eye such that a single image is perceived and that **diplopia** and **confusion** are not present. **Sensory fusion** does not necessary imply that **stereopsis** will be present.

fusion amplitude
Synonym of ***fusional reserve.***

fusion maldevelopment nystagmus syndrome
A form of **infantile onset nystagmus** that is induced or made worse by occlusion of either eye. Beat direction is towards the fixating eye, and **nystagmus amplitude** is greater when the fixating eye is in **abduction**. **Nystagmus waveform** has linear or decelerating slow phases. There are two types: **latent latent nystagmus** and **manifest latent nystagmus**. There is also **naso-temporal optokinetic asymmetry**. *Acronym is* ***FMNS.*** *Synonym is* ***latent nystagmus.***

fusional convergence
Convergence stimulated by the need for visual **fusion**.

fusional reserve
The amount of prism that can be tolerated after a **heterophoria** is compensated for. *Acronym is FR. Synonym is **fusion amplitude**.*

fusional vergence
The amount of prism that can be tolerated before **diplopia** occurs in **fusional reserve** testing. *Synonym is **break point**.*

FVFDC
*Acronym of **fused vergence fixation disparity curve**.*

G

GA
Acronym of ***geographic atrophy.***

GABA
Acronym of γ*-aminobutyric acid.*

Gabor patch
A sine wave grating stimulus with equal luminance to its background, visible over a circular area. Often used in **psychophysics** experiments.

Galilean telescope
Smaller than a **Keplerian telescope**; composed of two lenses. Little ocular relief, and blurred at the periphery of the image. **Exit pupil** is within the system. *Synonym is* ***dioptric telescope.***

gamut
The complete set of colours present in an image.

gangliocyte
Synonym of ***retinal ganglion cell.***

ganglion cell
Synonym of ***retinal ganglion cell.***

ganglion cell layer
Layer of the retina between the **nerve fibre layer** and the **inner plexiform layer** containing **ganglion cell** nuclei and displaced **amacrine cells**. *Acronym is GCL.*

Ganzfeld bowl
An illuminated bowl that a patient can put their head into to achieve full-field stimulation. Used in **electro-oculography** to reduce error.

gas permeable lens
Synonym of ***rigid gas permeable.***

GAT
Acronym of Goldmann applanation tonometry.

gaze
The direction in which the **fovea**(e) are pointing.

gaze evoked nystagmus
End-point nystagmus that does not cease after a short time. May include **rebound nystagmus**. Caused by a cerebellar issue. *Synonym is* ***gaze paretic nystagmus.***

gaze paretic nystagmus
*Synonym of **gaze evoked nystagmus**.*

GCL
*Acronym of **ganglion cell layer**.*

GDP
Acronym of guanosine diphosphate.

gegenrücke
*Synonym of **square-wave intrusion**.*

G

gelatinous drop-like dystrophy
Progressive **corneal** dystrophy causing subepithelial nodules, often with **neovascularisation**. *Synonym is **primary familial amyloidosis**.*

general fibrosis syndrome
Mechanical restriction due to fibrosed **extraocular muscles**. **Ptosis** and downwardly deviated eyes. Patients often have an elevated chin **abnormal head posture**.

generalised cones
Cylindrical shapes that the **Marr and Nishihara object recognition model** theorises all perceptual objects are broken into.

geniculocortical pathway
The pathway in the brain to the **visual cortex** via the **lateral geniculate nucleus** (90% of **ganglion cells** lead here). *Synonym is **retinogeniculocortical pathway**.*

geographic age-related macular degeneration
*Synonym of **dry age-related macular degeneration**.*

geographic atrophy
Large, well-defined areas of atrophy. A sign of **dry age-related macular degeneration**. *Acronym is **GA**.*

geometric inset
The horizontal distance from the **optical centre** for distance of a bifocal to the geometric centre of the reading **addition**.

geometric optics
The area of study concerning light, and methods for calculating its path, **vergence**, and **aberrations**.

geons
Thirty-six unambiguous shapes that, according to **Biederman's recognition by components theory**, form all perceptual objects.

gerontoxon
*Synonym of **arcus senilis**.*

gestalt psychology
Top-down theory of visual processing suggesting that perception is holistic.

GH
Acronym of general health.

ghost vessels
Previously active blood vessels that no longer contain blood. Tend to have abrupt endings and may spontaneously regress. When seen in the **cornea**, distinguish from nerve fibres which never regress and do not terminate abruptly.

GI
Acronym of gastrointestinal.

giant cell arteritis
Rare condition usually affecting 65–85-year-old women. Causes **arteritic anterior ischaemic optic neuropathy**. **Jaw claudication**, tender scalp, **polymyalgia rheumatica**. Not all signs may be present. *Synonym is **temporal arteritis**.*

giant papillary conjunctivitis
Contact lens induced papillary conjunctivitis in which the **papillae** are >1 mm in size. *Acronym is **GPC**.*

Giles–Archer colour perception unit
A **lantern test**.

glands of Krause
Mucous glands located at the **fornix**. One of the accessory **lacrimal glands**. *Synonym is **Krause glands**.*

glands of Wolfring
One of the accessory **lacrimal glands**. *Synonym is **Wolfring glands**.*

glands of Zeis
*Synonym of **Zeis glands**.*

glass blower's cataract
*Synonym of **heat cataract**.*

glaucoma
A group of conditions characterised by progressive damage of the optic nerve, usually due to high **intraocular pressure**.

glaucoma hemifield test
On a **perimetry** printout, a statistical test that compares vertically symmetrical regions of **visual field** either side of the **raphé** in areas known to be affected by **glaucoma**.

glaucomatocyclitic crisis
Synonym of ***Posner–Schlossman syndrome****.*

glaukomflecken
Anterior subcapsular or capsular **lens opacity** due to epithelial damage; sign of previous acute **closed angle glaucoma** attack.

G

glial cells
Provide support and structure to nerve cells.

glioma
Cancer of a nerve.

glissade
The fast drift back to **fixation** following a **dysmetric saccade**.

globe
Refers to the relatively spherical structure of the eye as a whole. *Synonym is* ***eyeball****.*

globulins
Protein in the blood involved in transport.

glucosuria
Excretion of sugar in urine in diabetics that leads to bodily fluid imbalances.

glutamate
Neurotransmitter used by **bipolar cells**, **ganglion cells**, and photoreceptors.

glycated haemoglobin test
Test that monitors average glucose levels over a long period of time.

glycation
Sugar bonding to protein or **lipid** without the use of an enzyme.

glycocalyx
Long chain of **glycoproteins**. Present at the base of the **mucous layer** of the tear film.

glycoprotein
Protein joined to carbohydrate.

glycosaminoglycan
Long unbranched polysaccharide.

GMP
Acronym of guanosine monophosphate.

gnosanopsia
The awareness of the presence of a visual stimulus, without being able to discriminate form. *Opposite of* **agnosopsia**.

gnosopsia
The normal condition of having conscious awareness of vision, and being able to make discriminations about visual stimuli. Compare with **anopsia**, **agnosopsia**, and **gnosanopsia**.

goblet cells
Mucus secreting cells.

Goldmann tonometer
Uses a probe with a diameter of 3.06 mm which presses against the **cornea** to estimate **intraocular pressure**. Considered to be the gold standard in **tonometry**.

Goldmann–Weekers dark adaptometer
A type of dark adaptometer that is no longer produced.

Golgi apparatus
Adds sugar residue to proteins; packages and sends proteins away to destinations.

Golgi tendon organ
Sensory receptor located at the insertion of muscles into tendons.

Golgi tendon organ reflex
Causes relaxation of muscle to prevent damage during excessive contraction. *Synonym is* ***inverse stretch reflex***.

gonioscopy
Examination of the apex of the chamber angle with a goniolens.

Gottlieb visual field awareness system
An **expansion prism** system consisting of a single prism that is placed temporal to the **optical centre**, with the base in the direction of field loss.

GPC
Acronym of ***giant papillary conjunctivitis***.

gradient method
Method of calculating **accommodative convergence:accommodation ratio.** Formula: (angle between eyes with a spherical lens in place minus the angle without the lens) divided by the power of the lens used. **Eso** deviations should be input as a positive value and **exo** as negative. For an accurate result, **dynamic retinoscopy** should be performed to account for any **accommodative lag** or **accommodative lead**.

G

Gram staining
Stain used to differentiate bacteria into two distinct groups – **Gram-positive** and **Gram-negative**.

Gram-negative
Bacteria that do not stain using **Gram staining**.

Gram-positive
Bacteria that stain using **Gram staining**.

Granit–Harper law
Critical flicker fusion frequency that increases linearly with the log of the stimulus size.

G

Granit's component analysis
Splits **electroretinography** data into PI, PII, and PIII.

granular dystrophy
Corneal stromal dystrophy: three types. Crumb-like appearance. All are treated by **penetrating keratoplasty**.

granular dystrophy type I
Onset 1st decade with recurrent **corneal erosion**s.

granular dystrophy type II
Onset 4th–5th decade with or without recurrent **corneal erosion**s.

granular dystrophy type III
Onset old age, without recurrent **corneal erosion**s. *Synonym is* ***Avellino dystrophy***.

grating acuity
The **visual acuity** for resolution of the direction of a regularly spaced grating. Easier to resolve for horizontal/vertical orientations. Often better than letter acuity as can see the interference pattern.

Graves' disease
Systemic condition, causing **hyperthyroidism**. *Synonym is* ***Basedow–Graves disease***.

Graves' ophthalmopathy
Synonym of ***thyroid eye disease***.

Graves' orbitopathy
Synonym of ***thyroid eye disease***.

Green's formula
Depth of focus of the eye {in dioptres} = 7.03/(**visual acuity** {in cycles/°} * **pupil** size {in mm}).

grey matter
Concentration of nerve cell bodies. Found centrally in the spinal cord and the outer layers of the brain.

Grönblad–Strandberg syndrome
Pseudoxanthoma elasticum and **angioid streaks** when they present together.

Grundy's visibility indicator
Chart used to determine suitability of lighting levels in a home environment for a patient's visual capabilities when undertaking a near task. The visibility of dots of varying **contrast** and **spatial frequency** are compared in the clinic to the home environment. If there is a discrepancy, lighting at home should be improved.

gt
Abbreviation of ***gutta****.*

GTP
Acronym of guanosine triphosphate.

gtt
Abbreviation of ***guttae****.*

guanylate cyclase
Synthesises cyclic guanosine monophosphate.

guanylate cyclase activating protein
Activated by a decrease in the concentration of calcium. Activates **guanylate cyclase**.

Gullstrand photokeratoscope
A type of **cornea**l topographer – uses a **Placido disc** and camera.

Gunn's sign
Synonym of ***nipping****.*

gutta
Drop (medical). *Abbreviation is* ***gt****. Plural is* ***guttae****.*

guttae
Plural of ***gutta****.*

guttata
Permanent collagen deposits at posterior **Descemet's membrane**. Appear as dark spots.

Gx
Abbreviation of glasses.

gyrate atrophy

Inherited pigment dysfunction disease. Causes **nyctalopia** and circular patches of pigment in the mid-peripheral **fundus**.

gyrus

Outward bulge of the brain.

H

H
Abbreviation of ***hyperphoria****.*

h.s.
Acronym of hora somni (at bedtime).

H&S
Acronym of history and symptoms.

HA
Acronym of headache/health authority.

HAART
Acronym of ***highly active antiretroviral therapy****.*

haemolytic glaucoma
Glaucoma caused by blood debris clogging the **trabecular meshwork.** May occur following an **intragel haemorrhage** or **preretinal haemorrhage**.

haemoptysis
Coughing up of blood.

Haidinger's brush
Entoptic phenomenon causing the appearance of yellow haze in the **macular** region upon a bright blue background when viewed by a rotating polarised filter, due to the crystal-like structure of **xanthophyll** pigment.

Haller's layer
The outermost, larger of the **choroid**al blood vessel layers.

hallucination
Any sensory perception occurring without a physical stimulus.

Halmagyi–Curthoys head impulse test
Clinical test of the **vestibulo-ocular reflex** in which the head is moved rapidly from side to side. If the test fails, the patient's eyes deviate towards the direction of the thrust, followed (usually) by a corrective **saccade**.

Hannover's canal
The circular space between the two dense portions of the **zonules of Zinn**. *Synonym is* ***canal of Hannover****.*

haploscope
A device that presents two different images to each eye. **Synoptophore**s and **amblyoscope**s are examples.

haptic lens
Synonym of ***scleral contact lens.***

HARC
Acronym of ***harmonious anomalous retinal correspondence.***

hard drusen
Small, nodular, yellow-white spots found at the **fundus**. A few can be normal in the periphery due to age. *Synonym is* ***nodular drusen.***

hard exudates
Lipoprotein and **lipid**-filled macrophages between the **inner plexiform layer** and **inner nuclear layer** of the retina, due to oedema. *Acronym is HE.*

harmonious anomalous retinal correspondence
Anomalous retinal correspondence in which the subjective angle of deviation is zero. Can lead to a form of binocular vision in patients with **strabismus**. *Acronym is HARC.*

Hart chart
A pair of **optotype** charts, shown at 40 cm and 3 m. The patient reads lines from alternating charts, as a measure of **accommodative facility**.

Hasner's fold
Synonym of ***Hasner's valve.***

Hasner's valve
Fold of mucosa often found at the end of the **nasolacrimal duct**. *Synonym is* ***Hasner's fold.***

Hassall–Henle bodies
Guttata in the peripheral **cornea**; seen in all individuals.

Hassenstein–Reichardt detector
Synonym of ***Reichardt detector.***

Hb
Abbreviation of haemoglobin.

HbA1C
Abbreviation of glycated haemoglobin.

HBP
Acronym of ***Heimann–Bielschowsky phenomenon.***

HE
*Acronym of **hard exudates**.*

head tilt test
*Synonym of **Bielschowsky head tilt test**.*

head-mounted display
A display device worn on the head to facilitate **extended reality**. *Acronym is **HMD**.*

headache
Typically categorised as either **primary headache** or **secondary headache**.

heat cataract
Cataract caused by exposure to infra-red light. *Synonym is **glass blower's cataract**.*

heavy eye syndrome
Hypotropia caused by abnormal **lateral rectus** position due to the weight of high **myopia**. *Synonym is **progressive esotropia fixus**.*

Heijl–Krakau technique
In **perimetry**, providing a target where the patient's physiological blind spot should be. Tests if the patient is maintaining good **fixation**.

Heimann–Bielschowsky phenomenon
Monocular pendular vertical low frequency **nystagmus** seen in some patients with severe monocular vision loss.

helminth
A type of parasitic worm.

HEMA
Acronym of 2-Hydroxyethyl methacrylate.

hemeralopia
Reduced visual function under **photopic** conditions. Note: occasionally hemeralopia is used as a synonym for **nyctalopia**.

hemiachromatopsia
Cerebral achromatopsia affecting only one **hemifield**.

hemianopia
Loss of half the **visual field** with respect to vertical midline. *Synonym is **hemianopsia**.*

hemianopic line bisection error
Phenomenon whereby a patient with **hemianopia** will bisect horizontal lines with a bias towards their blind **hemifield**, even in the absence of **unilateral neglect**.

hemianopsia
Synonym of ***hemianopia.***

hemidesmosome
Connects **intermediate filaments** in the basal domain of epithelial cells to **laminal** cells.

hemidyschromatopsia
Cerebral dyschromatopsia affecting only one **hemifield.**

hemifield
Either the left or right half of the **visual field.**

H

hemifield neglect
Synonym of ***unilateral neglect.***

hemislide phenomenon
Diplopia due to no **fusion** due to no overlap of **visual fields**, e.g. in **bitemporal hemianopia** or similar.

hemispatial neglect
Synonym of ***unilateral neglect.***

Henle's fibre layer
The **outer plexiform layer** at the **macula.**

Henson screener
Type of electronic **perimeter** – uses multiple stimuli at suprathreshold.

Hering theory
Synonym of ***opponent theory.***

Hering's law of equal innervation
For **conjugate eye movements**, **contralateral synergists** receive equal innervation from the central nervous system.

Hermann grid
Visual illusion involving a grid of black squares; grey areas are seen at the intersections (due to **lateral inhibition**).

Hermansky–Pudlak syndrome
Rare genetic disorder. Causes **oculocutaneous albinism.**

herpes simplex keratitis
Causes a dendritic staining pattern. Caused by **herpes simplex virus type 1**. *Synonym is* ***herpetic keratitis.***

herpes simplex virus
Lies dormant in the ganglion of the trigeminal nerve. There are two types: **herpes simplex virus type 1** and herpes simplex virus type 2. *Acronym is **HSV**.*

herpes simplex virus type 1
Causes cold sores, **corneal ulcers**, **keratoconjunctivitis**. Often treated with aciclovir. *Acronym is **HSV-1**.*

herpes zoster
*Synonym of **shingles**.*

herpes zoster ophthalmicus
Shingles affecting the **ophthalmic nerve**.

herpetic keratitis
*Synonym of **herpes simplex keratitis**.*

Herrick plug
An intracanalicular **punctal** plug.

Hertel exophthalmometer
Device comprising rulers and mirrors used to measure the magnitude of **proptosis**.

HES
Acronym of hospital eye service.

Hess screen
Similar to **Lees screen** but with only one panel. Red and green threads and filters dissociate the eyes.

heterochromia
Different colour between irides or within the same iris. *Synonym is **heterochromia iridis**.*

heterochromia iridis
*Synonym of **heterochromia**.*

heteronymous diplopia
Right eye's image is perceived on the left side, left eye's image on the right (i.e. cross-eyed). *Synonym is **crossed diplopia**.*

heteronymous hemianopia
Loss of the opposite halves of vision in both eyes. Could be caused by pituitary tumour.

heteronymous retinal disparity
*Synonym of **crossed retinal disparity**.*

H

heterophoria
Latent deviation in the angle between the eyes; may become manifest in the absence of visual stimulus, with fatigue, intoxication, etc. *Synonym is **phoria**.*

heterophoria method
*Synonym of **phoria method**.*

heterotropia
*Synonym of **strabismus**.*

HFA
*Acronym of **Humphrey field analyser**.*

hiding Heidi
Contrast sensitivity test for children. Various **contrast** levels of a face; child has to choose the target with the face between a face or blank card. Test at one metre.

high blood pressure
*Synonym of **hypertension**.*

high threshold theory
Theory that suggests stimuli are only perceived if their intensity crosses a given threshold. Does not account for **false alarms**. Superseded by **signal detection theory**.

highly active antiretroviral therapy
Describes when multiple antiretroviral drugs are used at once. *Acronym is **HAART**.*

hilum
In anatomy, any **depression** or pit to which structures attach.

hippus
A low-amplitude oscillation of **pupil** size (approx 1.4 Hz) seen in normals, especially in the young or **photopic** conditions.

Hirschberg test
Performed by shining a light in the patient's eyes and observing where the light reflects off the **corneas**. Used to estimate the magnitude of a **strabismus**. 1 mm of deviation roughly equates to a 7° angular deviation.

HIV
Acronym of human immunodeficiency virus.

HIV retinal microangiopathy
*Synonym of **AIDS retinopathy**.*

HIV retinopathy
*Synonym of **AIDS retinopathy**.*

HLA
Acronym of human leukocyte antigen.

HM
Acronym of hand movements.

HMD
Acronym of ***head-mounted display.***

hMT+
Refers to areas **MT, MST,** and neighbouring motion-sensitive **extrastriate cortex** in humans.

HOA
Acronym of higher-order aberration.

H

Hoffstetter formula
Expected **amplitude of accommodation** of an individual = 18.5 – 0.3 × age of patient.

Hollenhorst plaque
Bright deposit of cholesterol found at arteriolar bifurcations in the **fundus**. *Synonym is cholesterol emboli.*

Holmes–Adie tonic pupil
Synonym of ***Adie's pupil.***

Holmes stereoscope
Device consisting of two images, separated by a **septum**. Binocularity is measured with varying prism/lenses.

Holmes–Wright lantern
A **lantern test** that has been discontinued but is occasionally used on appeal by British armed forces if test CP 2 is failed.

homatropine
An antimuscarinic **cycloplegic**.

homocystinuria
Hereditary metabolic disorder, causing high **myopia** and **ectopia lentis**.

homonymous
On the same side; in the context of **visual field** defects, refers to the visual loss being in the same (left or right) side of the vertical midline of each eye.

homonymous congruous defect
Visual field defects in each eye which are **homonymous** and similarly shaped.

homonymous hemianopia
Loss of same half of vision in both eyes. Caused by **stroke** or tumour posterior to the **optic chiasm**.

homonymous retinal disparity
Synonym of ***uncrossed retinal disparity.***

homunculus
A theoretical model of the human body that proportionately represents the amount of motor/sensory cortex receptors devoted to each effector of the body.

hordeolum
Infection (usually staphylococcal) of a gland or follicle of the **eyelid**, often after a blockage. Usually painful. Classified as an **external hordeolum** or **internal hordeolum**.

horizontal cell
Cell type present in the **outer plexiform layer**, which connects photoreceptors together, to create **receptive fields**.

horizontal saccade palsy
Eyes deviated to side of **lesion**. Patient cannot make **saccade**s but can use **smooth pursuit** to move eyes towards a target.

horizontal visible iris diameter
Measurement used for contact lens fitting, of the visible size of the iris across the horizontal meridian, measured at the **cornea**. **Rigid gas permeable** total diameter should be 1.5–2 mm smaller than this. *Acronym is* ***HVID***.

Horner–Trantas dots
White dots at the **limbus**; epithelial cells and eosinophils. A sign of **vernal keratoconjunctivitis**.

Horner's muscle
Part of the **orbicularis oculi**. Contracts during a blink, squeezing the **lacrimal sac**.

Horner's pupil
Synonym of ***Horner's syndrome.***

Horner's syndrome
Ptosis, **miosis**, facial **anhidrosis**, cluster headaches, poor **pupil** reflexes. Due to sympathetic nervous system **lesion**. *Synonyms are* ***Bernard–Horner syndrome*** *and* ***Horner's pupil.***

horopter
Imaginary plane made from all the points of **retinal correspondence**.

horseshoe break
Synonym of ***horseshoe tear.***

horseshoe tear
A U-shaped retinal tear. *Synonym is* ***horseshoe break.***

Howell phoria card
Tool to measure subjective **heterophoria**. A vertical prism dissociates the eyes, and the patient is asked which number an arrow points to. Distance and near versions available.

HRT
Acronym of Heidelberg retinal tomography.

HSV
Acronym of ***herpes simplex virus.***

HSV-1
Acronym of ***herpes simplex virus type 1.***

Hudson–Stähli line
Orange iron deposition line seen on the **cornea** where the **eyelid**s meet; normal with age.

Humphrey field analyser
A device for measuring central **visual field**s – considered the gold standard in modern **perimetry**. *Acronym is* ***HFA.***

Humphriss fogging method
One eye is fogged with a positive lens, the other is left clear to allow a binocular **refraction** to be balanced through fine adjustments in the prescription in the unfogged eye.

hundred day glaucoma
Neovascular glaucoma secondary to a **central retinal vein occlusion.**

Hutchinson pupil
Unilateral **dilation** due to compression of the **oculomotor nerve** by space occupying **lesion** on that side. Patient in a coma.

Hutchinson sign
Involvement of the tip of the nose in shingles. Associated with **herpes zoster ophthalmicus**.

Hutchinson's freckle
Synonym of ***lentigo maligna.***

Huygen's principle
Each point on a wavefront is the source of wavelets.

HVID
Acronym of ***horizontal visible iris diameter.***

H

Hx
Abbreviation of history.

hyalocyte
A phagocytic cell found in the **vitreous humour**.

hyaloid artery
Artery that supplies the anterior eye during embryological development. *Synonyms are **canal of Stilling**, **hyaloid vessel**, and **Stilling's canal**.*

hyaloid canal
The area in which the **hyaloid artery** develops during foetal growth.

hyaloid vessel
*Synonym of **hyaloid artery**.*

hyaloideocapsular ligament
*Synonym of **Wieger's ligament**.*

hyaluronan
A **glycosaminoglycan** present in the **vitreous humour**. Maintains the osmotic balance of the vitreous. *Synonym is **hyaluronic acid**.*

hyaluronic acid
*Synonym of **hyaluronan**.*

hydrocephalus
Accumulation of cerebrospinal fluid in the brain. Causes increased intracranial pressure. Congenital. Can be due to damage to the **abducens nerve**.

hydrophthalmos
*Synonym of **buphthalmos**.*

hydrops
Dua's layer breaks, leading to **corneal oedema** and scarring. Causes sudden vision loss. Occurs in **keratoconus** and **Pellucid marginal degeneration**.

hydroxychloroquine
An analogue of **chloroquine** with similar ocular effects.

Hyper
*Abbreviation of **hyperphoria**.*

Hyper(T)
*Abbreviation of intermittent **hypertropia**.*

hyperacuity
The ability to detect stimulus misalignment above expected **visual acuity**. Applies to **vernier acuity**.

hyperaemia
Increased blood flow to a part of the body. In the eye, causes redness of vessels. *Synonym is **injection**.*

hypercapnia
High carbon dioxide concentration in solution (can be used to describe tears if applicable).

hypercholesterolaemia
High cholesterol.

hypercolumn
A 1 mm column through the **primary visual cortex** containing cells specific to all orientations and ocular dominances for a given retinal locus.

hypercomplex cell
*Synonym of **end-stopped cell**.*

hyperglycemia
High glucose levels. Sign of diabetes.

hypermetric saccade
A **saccade** that 'over-shoots' its intended **location**.

hypermetropia
*Synonym of **hyperopia**.*

hyperocular lenses
Highly positive spectacle lenses designed for use as magnifiers.

hyperope
An individual with **hyperopia**.

hyperopia
The condition in which parallel light is focused behind the retina when **accommodation** is relaxed. Individuals often have a shorter than average axial length and a shallow optic cup. *Synonyms are **farsightedness** and **hypermetropia**.*

hyperphoria
Vertical **heterophoria**. The eye with the resting point higher than the other is considered hyperphoric. *Abbreviations are **H** and **Hyper**.*

hyperplasia
Describes an organ that is too large because there are too many cells – the size of cells is normal.

hyperreflexia
Excessive reflex responses; e.g. **twitch**ing.

HyperT
Abbreviation of ***hypertropia*****.**

hypertelorism
Describes a large **interpupillary distance**.

hypertension
High arterial blood pressure. *Synonym is* ***high blood pressure*****.**

hypertensive choroidopathy
Occurs in severe **hypertension. Retinal pigment epithelium** lesions, **Elschnig spots, Siegrist streaks.**

hypertensive retinopathy
Oedema, **exudates, flame haemorrhages, focal intraretinal periarteriolar transudates, intraretinal microvascular abnormalities, macular star, copper wiring/silver wiring.**

hyperthyroidism
Decreased weight, increased metabolism, increased blood pressure, increased temperature, sweating, fatigue, **palpitations**. May cause **thyroid eye disease**.

hypertonic
High salt content.

hypertrichosis
Trichomegaly and/or **polytrichosis**.

hypertrophy
Describes an organ that is too large because the cells are too large (the number of cells is normal).

hypertropia
A manifest ocular deviation in an upwards direction. *Abbreviation is* ***HyperT*****.**

hyperviscosity
Thick blood; slow flow. **Cotton wool spots**, haemorrhages, venous **dilation**, and tortuosity. Complication of **leukaemia**.

hyphaema
Blood in the **anterior chamber**.

hypnic headache
A form of **primary headache**, typically affecting middle-aged to elderly patients. Headaches wake patient from sleep.

Hypo
Abbreviation of ***hypophoria****.*

Hypo(T)
Abbreviation of intermittent ***hypotropia****.*

hypoaesthesia
Reduced sensitivity to pain/touch/temperature. In reference to the **cornea**, indicates reduced **corneal touch threshold**.

hypofibrinogenemia
Very little **fibrinogen**, therefore little clotting.

hypoglycemia
When a diabetic drinks alcohol on an empty stomach or has too much insulin. Causes **palpitations**.

hypometric saccade
A **saccade** that 'under-shoots' its intended **location**.

hypophoria
Vertical **heterophoria**. The eye with the resting point lower than the other is considered hypophoric. *Abbreviation is* ***Hypo****.*

hypoplasia
Incomplete development of an organ or body part. *Synonym is* ***dysgenesis****.*

hypopyon
Pus in the **anterior chamber**, as a result of infection. Settles in the bottom of the anterior chamber, often can be seen through the **cornea** as a white deposit.

HypoT
Abbreviation of ***hypotropia****.*

hypotony
Intraocular pressure ≤5 mmHg. Can cause **choroidal folds**.

hypotropia
A manifest ocular deviation in a downwards direction. *Abbreviation is* ***HypoT****.*

hypoxia
Deprivation of oxygen.

hypromellose
A viscoliser component of many artificial tears.

hysterical blindness
Reduced vision entirely due to psychological reasons.

hysterical flutter
Synonym of ***voluntary nystagmus****.*

hysterical nystagmus
Synonym of ***voluntary nystagmus****.*

H

hysterical visual fields
A nonsense **visual field** plot, produced by malingerers, whether deliberate or not. In Goldmann fields, the plot is usually spiral-shaped; with the **Bjerrum screen**, often the same ring is seen regardless of distance and with **Humphrey field analysers/Henson screeners**, supposed field loss tends to be random.

I

I
Abbreviation of luminous intensity.

I&C
Acronym of ***incision and curatage****.*

I&R
Acronym of insertion and removal.

IAP
Acronym of inhibitor of apoptosis protein.

iatrogenic
Describes an effect (good or bad) caused by medical error.

ICE
Acronym of ***iridocorneal endothelial syndrome****.*

ICG
Acronym of ***indocyanine green****.*

ICP
Acronym of intracranial pressure.

ICRS
Acronym of ***intra-corneal ring segments****.*

ICS
Acronym of intermittent convergent strabismus.

ID
Acronym of intellectual difficulty.

IDD
Acronym of insulin-dependent diabetes.

IDDM
Acronym of insulin-dependent diabetes mellitus.

idiopathic
Of an unknown cause.

idiopathic central serous retinopathy
Synonym of ***central serous retinopathy.***

idiopathic congenital nystagmus
Synonym of ***idiopathic infantile nystagmus.***

idiopathic full-thickness macular hole
Occurs most often in elderly women. Vitreal contraction causes a **retinal detachment**; a pseudo-operculum forms and disappears. The condition is traditionally thought to occur in four stages: **vitreomacular traction**; small hole; medium hole; large hole without adhesion of the **vitreous**. Treatment is by **vitrectomy** or **ocriplasmin** injection.

idiopathic infantile nystagmus
Infantile nystagmus in which no cause for the **nystagmus** can be diagnosed. *Acronym is IIN. Synonyms are* ***congenital idiopathic nystagmus, idiopathic congenital nystagmus,*** *and* ***idiopathic motor nystagmus.***

I

idiopathic intracranial hypertension
Increased intracranial pressure without obvious cause. Typically affects young obese women. *Acronym is* ***IIH****. Synonyms are* ***benign intracranial hypertension*** *and* ***pseudotumour cerebri.***

idiopathic motor nystagmus
Synonym of ***idiopathic infantile nystagmus.***

idiopathic orbital inflammatory disease
Pseudotumour. Oedema of the upper lateral **eyelid**. Downward and inward **globe** displacement.

idiopathic premacular fibrosis
Synonym of ***epiretinal membrane.***

idiopathic vitritis
Inflammation of the **vitreous humour**. Causes oedema, **floaters**, and blurred vision. Occurs in older patients, usually female.

IDS
Acronym of intermittent divergent strabismus.

IIH
Acronym of ***idiopathic intracranial hypertension.***

IIN
Acronym of ***idiopathic infantile nystagmus.***

illuminance
Luminous flux per unit area (amount of light hitting a surface). Measured in **lux**. *Synonym is* ***illumination.***

illumination
*Synonym of **illuminance**.*

ILM
*Acronym of **inner limiting membrane**.*

Imbert–Fick law
An external force against a sphere is equal to the pressure in the sphere multiplied by the area applanated.

implicit time
The time from stimulus presentation until the peak of the electropotential component.

IN
*Acronym of **infantile nystagmus**.*

inattentional blindness
Completely missing something in the visual scene due to lack of attention.

INC
*Acronym of **interstitial nucleus of Cajal**.*

incidence
The probability that any individual will develop a disease over a given time period. Compare with **prevalence**.

incision and curatage
Method of **chalazion** removal – opened surgically and drained. *Acronym is **I&C**.*

inclusion conjunctivitis
Type of **chlamydial conjunctivitis**. May be passed on during birth; can also be transmitted in swimming pools or on eye makeup.

incomitance
Condition in which the dissociated angle between the eyes is not maintained in all angles of **gaze**. *Adjective form is **incomitant**.*

incomitant
*Adjective form of **incomitance**.*

incongruous
Not similar.

increment threshold
In **psychophysics**, the smallest difference in intensity of two stimuli that can be perceived. *Synonyms are **difference threshold** and **just noticeable difference**.*

I

incycloduction
Monocular **intorsion**.

incyclophoria
Latent eye deviation in which the top pole of the eye rotates in the nasal direction.

incyclorotation
Monocular eye movement in which the upper pole of the eye rotates nasally. *Synonym is* ***intorsion****. Verb form is* ***intort****.*

incyclotropia
Manifest eye deviation in which the top pole of the eye rotates in the nasal direction.

incyclovergence
Binocular eye movement in which the upper **cornea**l poles of both eyes rotate inward.

I

index myopia
Myopia induced by a change in the **refractive index** of intraocular structures. This often refers to the myopic shift seen in **cataract** progression.

index of refraction
Synonym of ***refractive index****.*

indirect goniolens
Uses mirrors to overcome total internal reflection.

indocyanine green
Dye used in angiography. Used to assess **choroid**al circulation; does not leak like **sodium fluorescein**. *Acronym is* ***ICG****.*

induced motion
Perceived motion of one object caused by real movement of another adjacent object.

infantile esotropia syndrome
A **constant esotropia** without an accommodative element with size >30 **prism dioptre**s and onset within the first six months of life. Often occurs in conjunction with **fusion maldevelopment nystagmus syndrome**, **dissociated vertical deviation**, overactive **inferior oblique**s, and an **abnormal head posture**. *Synonym is* ***congenital strabismus syndrome****.*

infantile nystagmus
Nystagmus that develops in the first six months of life, in response (usually) to a visual system abnormality. It is known to occur in the absence of known pathology (**idiopathic infantile nystagmus**), although it is possible in these cases that an abnormality remains undiagnosed. There is often a **null zone** at which the oscillations are minimised. *Acronym is* ***IN****. Synonyms are* ***congenital nystagmus*** *and* ***infantile nystagmus syndrome****.*

infantile nystagmus syndrome
Synonym of ***infantile nystagmus****.*

infantile onset nystagmus
Any form of **nystagmus** that presents in the first few months of life, unless caused by a condition causing **acquired nystagmus** within that time. Includes **fusion maldevelopment nystagmus syndrome**, **spasmus nutans**, and **infantile nystagmus**.

infarction
Artery blocked by an obstruction, causing necrosis.

infectious keratitis
*Synonym of **microbial infiltrative keratitis**.*

inferior arcuate stain
Sodium fluorescein staining pattern seen as an arc at the inferior **cornea**, caused by high water content soft contact lenses drawing water out of the cornea. *Synonym is **smile stain**.*

inferior frontal eye fields
Part of the **frontal eye fields** involved in **saccades** and **smooth pursuit**.

inferior oblique
One of the six **extraocular muscles**. Originates at the antero-medial **orbit**al floor, passes around the inferior **globe**, and inserts at the supero-temporal globe. Contraction causes **extorsion** (primarily), with **elevation** and **abduction**. Innervated by the **ipsilateral oculomotor nerve**. *Acronym is **IO**.*

inferior rectus
One of the six **extraocular muscles**. Originates at the **annulus of Zinn** and inserts at the infero-nasal **globe**. Contraction causes **depression** (primarily), with **extorsion** and **adduction**. Innervated by the **ipsilateral oculomotor nerve**.

inferotemporal cortex
Part of the brain selective to complex features – some areas specifically to face patterns. The area where vision interacts with **visual memory**. *Acronym is **IT**.*

infiltrate
Extra material in tissue spaces or cells. If contact lens related, often seen in the peripheral **cornea**.

inflammation
A non-specific response to tissue injury. Causes redness, swelling, heat, and pain.

infraduction
Monocular **depression**. *Synonym is **deorsumduction**.*

infranuclear neurogenic paralytic strabismus
Strabismus caused by **lesions** between the nerve nucleus and muscle, i.e. affecting the **oculomotor nerve**, **trochlear nerve**, or **abducens nerve**.

I

infraorbital
Below the **orbit**.

infraversion
Binocular eye movement: looking down.

inion
Knobbly ridge at the back of the skull – used as a reference point when attaching electrodes.

injection
Synonym of ***hyperaemia***.

INL
Acronym of ***inner nuclear layer***.

inner ciliary epithelium
Non-pigmented; constitutes the anterior continuation of the nervous part of the retina.

inner limiting membrane
Most anterior layer of the retina: **Müller cells** joined to the **vitreous humour** by fine collagen fibrils. Occasionally there are astrocytes present. *Acronym is* ***ILM***. *Synonym is* ***internal limiting membrane***.

inner nuclear layer
Layer of the retina containing the nuclei of **horizontal cells**, **bipolar cells**, **amacrine cells**, and **Müller cells**. *Acronym is* ***INL***.

inner plexiform layer
Layer of the retina at which **ganglion cells** synapse with **amacrine cells** and **bipolar cells**. *Acronym is* ***IPL***.

INO
Acronym of ***internuclear ophthalmoplegia***.

INS
Acronym of ***infantile nystagmus syndrome***.

integrated people-centred eye care
A model for organising eye care delivery which focuses on the needs of patients rather than the boundaries of service providers. There is a specific focus on linking different service providers together in order to streamline the patient journey. *Acronym is* ***IPEC***.

integrin
Protein that binds a cell to the extracellular matrix. Allows signal transduction between them.

inter-palpebral fit
Describes a contact lens that sits entirely between the **eyelids** when lids are normally open.

interblob
Areas of the **primary visual cortex** that don't stain with **cytochrome oxidase**. Areas containing orientation and **contrast**-specific **parvo cells**.

interface theory
Theory that visual perception is adapted to represent aspects of the world that are useful for evolutionary success, which may not necessarily be **veridical**. See also **depiction theory**.

interferometer
The instrument used in **interferometry**.

interferometry
Measuring the interference pattern produced by superposition of two waves.

interferon
Type of **cytokine** produced by the immune system to challenge pathogens.

interleukins
Group of **cytokines**.

intermediary tissue of Kuhnt
Separates the optic nerve from retinal layers.

intermediate filaments
Present in cytosol; very tough protein.

intermediate uvea
The posterior **ciliary body** and peripheral retina.

intermediate uveitis
Inflammation of the **intermediate uvea**.

internal hordeolum
A **hordeolum** affecting the **meibomian glands**.

internal limiting membrane
Synonym of ***inner limiting membrane***.

International Society for Clinical Electrophysiology of Vision
International group for agreement on standard protocols for clinical uses of **electroretinography**, **electro-oculography**, and **visual evoked potentials**. *Acronym is* ***ISCEV***.

International Society for Clinical Eye Tracking
International group for agreement on standard protocols for clinical uses of **eye trackers**. *Acronym is* ***ISCET***.

interneuron
A neuron that connects other neurons to one another.

internuclear neurogenic paralytic strabismus
Due to a **lesion** of the **medial longitudinal fasciculus**.

internuclear ophthalmoplegia
Mismatch in pulse and step signals caused by **lesion** of the ipsilateral **medial longitudinal fasciculus**. Absent **adduction** with ataxia **nystagmus** in the abducting eye. Often **exotropia**. *Acronym is **INO**.*

interpupillary distance
The distance between the centres of the **pupils**. *Acronyms are **IPD** and **PD**. Synonym is **pupillary distance**.*

interstitial nucleus of Cajal
The **neural integrator** for vertical and torsional eye movements. Situated in the **mesencephalic reticular formation**. *Acronym is **INC**.*

interstripe
In **V2**, part of the **parvocellular pathway** (but not colour-specific). Sensitive to orientation. *Synonym is **pale stripe**.*

intorsion
*Synonym of **incyclorotation**.*

intort
*Verb form of **incyclorotation**.*

intra-corneal ring segments
Semi-circular implant put into the **cornea** to treat mild **myopia**. Usually only used in in **keratoconus**. *Acronym is **ICRS**.*

intractable diplopia
Diplopia that shows no **adaptation** to any attempted treatment with lenses or prisms.

intraepithelial neoplasia
Conjunctival tumour: similar to **pterygia**; vascular, often in the elderly. Rarely malignant.

intrafusal muscle fibres
The muscle fibres of muscle spindles.

intragel haemorrhage
Haemorrhage into the **vitreous humour**. *Synonym is **vitreous haemorrhage**.*

intraLASIK
Femtosecond LASIK when an intralase laser is used.

intraocular
Inside or within the eye.

intraocular lens
Any type of false lens that is implanted inside the eye. *Acronym is **IOL**.*

intraocular muscles
The **sphincter pupillae, dilator pupillae**, and **ciliary muscle**.

intraocular pressure
The pressure within the eye. Measured by **tonometry**, and expressed in mmHg. *Acronym is **IOP**.*

intraretinal fluid
Fluid found above the photoreceptors, often as a result of **wet age-related macular degeneration**.

intraretinal microvascular abnormalities
Dilation of capillaries inside the retina. Occurs in **diabetic retinopathy** and **hypertensive retinopathy**. *Acronym is **IRMA**.*

intravitreal
Injection directly into the **vitreous**.

intrinsic activity
How well a drug elicits a response after it has bound to receptors.

intrinsic factor
Produced by parietal cells. Involved in absorption of vitamin B12.

intrinsic grey
*Synonym of **intrinsic light**.*

intrinsic light
Entoptic phenomenon: light perceived in complete darkness due to neural noise in photoreceptors. *Synonyms are **eigengrau**, **eigenlicht**, and **intrinsic grey**.*

intumescent cataract
A **lens opacity** which has swollen with fluid.

invasins
Secreted by bacteria to trigger host cell's phagocytic reflexes so that bacteria can enter.

inverse square law
Halving the distance from lamp to object quadruples the **illumination**.

I

inverse stretch reflex
Synonym of ***Golgi tendon organ reflex****.*

involutional sclerosis
Replacement **fibrosis** of blood vessels: the more that has occurred (with ageing), the less narrowing of vessels will occur in **hypertension**. Therefore, younger people show a greater amount of narrowing of vessels in hypertension.

IO
Acronym of ***inferior oblique****.*

iodopsin
Photopigment in cones, far less reactive to light than **rhodopsin**.

IOFB
Acronym of intraocular foreign body.

IOL
Acronym of ***intraocular lens****.*

IOM
Acronym of intraocular muscle.

ION
Acronym of ***anterior ischaemic optic neuropathy****.*

IOP
Acronym of ***intraocular pressure****.*

IP
Acronym of ingress protection.

IPD
Acronym of ***interpupillary distance****.*

IPEC
Acronym of ***integrated people-centred eye care****.*

IPL
Acronym of ***inner plexiform layer****.*

IPM
Acronym of interphotoreceptor matrix.

ipsilateral
Anatomical term. Means 'on the same side'.

ipsilateral antagonist
The **extraocular muscle** in the same eye that acts at same time as, and against, any given muscle.

ipsilesional
On the same hemisphere/**hemifield** as a brain **lesion**.

ipsipulsion
Lateropulsion in which patients have **hypermetric saccades** in the **ipsilateral** direction of, and **hypometric saccades** in the **contralateral** direction of, a brain lesion. The opposite of **contrapulsion**.

IR
*Acronym of **inferior rectus**/infra-red.*

iridectomy
A hole cut in the iris (usually to allow for **aqueous humour** drainage).

iridocorneal angle
*Synonym of **anterior chamber angle**.*

iridocorneal endothelial syndrome
Rare condition causing **corectopia**, **polycoria**, **Cogan–Reese syndrome**, progressive iris atrophy and **Chandler syndrome**. *Acronym is **ICE**.*

iridocyclitis
Combined **iritis** and **cyclitis**.

iridodialysis
Separation of the iris from the **ciliary body**. *Synonym is **coredialysis**.*

iris bombé
In **pupillary block**, **aqueous humour** build-up in the **posterior chamber** causes the iris to bulge out. May lead to **closed angle glaucoma**.

iris clip lens
A type of **phakic intraocular lens**, more commonly used in the 1960s. Causes the appearance of a square **pupil**, as the lens is attached to the iris. Don't use **mydriatics** on these, as it can cause the lens to dislodge.

iris coloboma
Always inferior, often nasal. May be just a notch or sector. Beware of **meridional amblyopia**.

iris root
*Synonym of **ciliary margin**.*

I

I

iritis
Inflammation of the iris.

Irlen syndrome
Synonym of ***visual stress.***

IRMA
Acronym of ***intraretinal microvascular abnormalities.***

Irvine–Gass syndrome
Cystoid macular oedema as a post-**cataract** surgery complication.

ISCET
Acronym of ***International Society for Clinical Eye Tracking.***

ISCEV
Acronym of ***International Society for Clinical Electrophysiology of Vision.***

ischaemia
Restriction in blood supply.

ischaemic diabetic maculopathy
Occluded capillaries, reduced **visual acuity** (despite normal appearance of **macula**), **hypoxia** (**neovascularisation** likely).

ischaemic retinal vein occlusion
Same as **non-ischaemic retinal vein occlusion** but more severe, less common, plus **neovascularisation** of the angle.

iseikonia
Having the same image size (usually referring to the images at the retinas); opposite of **aniseikonia**.

iseikonic lens
A lens with magnification but no power – could be used in **aniseikonia**, but contact lenses are usually a better option. *Synonym is* ***size lens.***

Ishihara colour plates
A test for screening for red-green colour defects. Does not pick up acquired (blue-yellow) defects.

ISNT rule
Indicates that, in reference to the **optic nerve head**, the inferior rim is larger than the superior, which in turn is larger than the nasal rim, with the temporal rim being the smallest.

isochromatic lenses
Lenses with an **equitint**.

isometropia
Both eyes having the same refractive error (or both having no refractive error).

isopter
A line joining points of equal threshold (sensitivity) derived from a **visual field** plot, i.e. a horizontal slice through the 'hill of vision'.

IT
Acronym of ***inferotemporal cortex****.*

IV
*Acronym of intermediate vision/intravenous/****intravitreal****.*

IVFA
Acronym of intravenous ***fluorescein angiography****.*

J

Jackson cross cylinder
A lens formed from two cylinders whose powers are numerically equal and of opposite sign, and whose axes are perpendicular to each other. Used to assess the cylindrical component of a patient's refractive state. *Acronym is* ***JCC****. Synonym is* ***cross cylinder****.*

JAM
Acronym of ***junctional adhesion molecule****.*

Javal–Schiotz keratometer
A type of **fixed doubling keratometer**.

jaw claudication
Pain on chewing.

jaw winking
Eyelid retraction is caused by jaw movement or swallowing. There is usually a **ptosis** in the affected eye. *Synonyms are* ***Marcus Gunn jaw winking*** *and* ***trigemino-oculomotor synkinesis****.*

JCC
Acronym of ***Jackson cross cylinder****.*

jelly bumps
Build-up of mucins, **lipid**, protein, and calcium, usually on a soft contact lens. More likely if the lens has a very high water content.

JIA
Acronym of ***juvenile idiopathic arthritis****.*

JND
Acronym of ***just noticeable difference****.*

Johnson's adherence syndrome
Extraocular muscles become stuck to something, e.g. each other (if they overlap). Causes mechanical restriction. *Synonym is* ***adherence syndrome****.*

Jones I test
Synonym of ***primary Jones test****.*

Jones II test
Synonym of ***secondary Jones test****.*

Jones test
Describes either the **primary Jones test** or **secondary Jones test**. *Synonyms are **dye disappearance test** and **fluorescein dye disappearance test**.*

Joubert syndrome
Rare genetic disorder. Causes **nystagmus** and **hypometric saccades/saccade initiation failure**.

junctional adhesion molecule
Found in tight junctions. *Acronym is **JAM**.*

just noticeable difference
*Synonym of **increment threshold**.*

juvenile arcus
Like **senile arcus** but occurring in younger individuals and is of clinical significance, as indicates **hypercholesterolaemia**.

juvenile chronic arthritis
*Synonym of **juvenile idiopathic arthritis**.*

juvenile idiopathic arthritis
Arthritis occurring before the age of 16; may be associated with **uveitis**. *Acronym is **JIA**. Synonyms are **juvenile chronic arthritis** and **Still's disease**.*

juvenile macular degeneration
*Synonym of **Stargardt disease**.*

juvenile optic atrophy
*Synonym of **dominant optic atrophy**.*

juvenile retinoschisis
Maculopathy: X-linked condition with young onset. **Electroretinography** is affected (reduced **b-wave**).

juxtacanicular tissue
Part of the **trabecular meshwork** against **Schlemm's canal**.

juxtapapillary
Describes something that is next to the **optic nerve head**.

K

K
*Abbreviation of **cornea/keratometry**.*

K-cells
*Abbreviation of **konio cells**.*

Kaposi sarcoma
Vascular tumour found on the **adnexa** in patients with AIDS.

kappa angle
*Synonym of **angle kappa**.*

Kasabach–Merritt syndrome
*Synonym of **thrombocytopenia**.*

Kayser–Fleischer ring
Copper deposits at the **Descemet's membrane** of the peripheral **cornea**. Indicative of **Wilson's disease.**

KCS
*Acronym of **keratoconjunctivitis sicca**.*

Kearns–Sayre syndrome
Retinitis pigmentosa, **progressive external ophthalmoplegia**, and complete heart block.

Keplerian telescope
Larger than a **Galilean telescope**, more ocular relief, wider field of view. The **exit pupil** is outside the optical system. *Synonym is **astronomical telescope**.*

keratic precipitates
Inflammatory cells from the iris/**ciliary body** (due to **iritis/cyclitis**) that adhere to the **corneal endothelium**. *Acronym is KP.*

keratitis
Inflammation of the **cornea**.

keratoacanthoma
Rare type of fast-growing **squamous cell carcinoma** often found on the lower **eyelid**. Rolled margins.

keratoconjunctivitis
Inflammation of both the **cornea** and **conjunctiva**.

keratoconjunctivitis sicca
Severe dry eye. *Acronym is **KCS**.*

keratoconus
Central **corneal ectasia**, causing bulging of the central cornea by pressure. Disorganised lamellæ in the **corneal stroma**. Causes **Vogt's striae**, **Rizzuti's sign**, **Fleischer ring**, and **Munson's sign**. Common in **Down syndrome**.

keratocytes
Form ~10% of the **corneal stroma**. Capable of **fibrillogenesis**. Maintain **corneal** fibril order. Transparent due to arrangement.

keratoglobus
Total **corneal ectasia**. Cause unknown. Can be associated with **Leber's congenital amaurosis**.

keratometer
A device that performs **keratometry**.

keratometry
The measurement of the curvature of the central **cornea**.

keratoplasty
Corneal transplant.

keratoprosthesis
A false **cornea**, indicated when the original cornea is so extensively damaged that a donor button would be rejected.

keratoscopy
A much more extensive type of **keratometry** done by a computer.

Kestenbaum surgery
Treatment to centralise the **null zone** of **nystagmus** by performing a **recession** on the pair of rectus muscles in the direction of the head turn and **resection** of the antagonists. *Synonym is **Anderson–Kestenbaum surgery**.*

ketoacidosis
Breakdown of fat for respiration. Occurs in type 1 diabetes when insulin levels are low and blood sugar levels are high.

kinetic occipital region
Brain area located close to **visual area middle temporal**. Processes kinetic boundaries (i.e. motion-defined edges). *Acronym is **KO**.*

kinetic perimetry
Perimetry in which a mobile stimulus is moved to plot the **visual field**, such as in Goldmann kinetic perimetry.

kinetic visual acuity
Visual acuity measurement for stimuli moving towards or away from the observer.

kinocilia
Hair-like projections in the **ampulla**e of the ear. Fluid movement causes them to bend, which excites or inhibits the **vestibular nerve** depending on the direction of movement.

Kjer's optic neuropathy
Synonym of ***dominant optic atrophy.***

knees of Wilbrand
The pathways followed by fibres from the nasal retinas at the **optic chiasm**. Two geniculate projections are present at each side of the **chiasm**; the anterior projection carries fibres from the inferior retina, and the posterior projection carries superior fibres. *Synonym is* ***Wilbrand's knees.***

KO
Acronym of ***kinetic occipital region.***

K

Kocher's sign
Frightened appearance due to **Dalrymple's sign**, especially when attentively fixating.

Koeppe lens
A **direct goniolens**.

Kollner's rule
Red-green colour vision problems are usually due to optic nerve disease, whilst blue-yellow colour vision problems are more likely to be due to retinal disease.

konio cells
Carry blue-yellow colour opponent info through the visual pathway. *Abbreviation is* ***K-cells.***

KP
Acronym of ***keratic precipitates.***

Krause glands
Synonym of ***glands of Krause.***

Krimsky test
An objective measure of **strabismus**. Like the **Hirschberg test**, a pen torch is used to obtain **corneal reflex**es. The strabismic eye is then balanced with a prism bar to find deviation.

Krukenberg spindle
Pigment deposition on the **corneal endothelium** in a vertical spindle pattern found in **pigment dispersion syndrome**.

L

L
Abbreviation of ***luminance****.*

L-cone
Abbreviation of red cone.

labyrinth
In the inner ear, the collective name for the **semicircular canals**, **ampullae**, and other aural vestibular apparatus. Disease of the labyrinths can cause **vestibular nystagmus.**

laceration
Irregular incision.

lacquer cracks
Ruptured **Bruch's membrane**. Shows as irregular yellow/white lines at **fundus**. Can be due to pathological **myopia**.

lacrimal artery
Supplies the **lacrimal gland** with blood. An early offshoot of the ophthalmic artery.

lacrimal bone
The most fragile bone in the face. Located at the front of the medial **orbit**.

lacrimal caruncle
The fleshy bulge of the medial **canthus**. Contains glands.

lacrimal fossa
Depression in the **lacrimal bone** where the **lacrimal sac** sits. A tumour here is called a **pleomorphic adenoma**.

lacrimal gland
Almond shaped two-lobed gland located in the superior temporal **orbit**. Secretes 90% of tears.

lacrimal layer
Synonym of ***aqueous layer****.*

lacrimal sac
The sac into which tears drain via the **puncta** and **canaliculi**. Leads to the **nasolacrimal duct**.

lacrimation
Crying or tearing.

L

lactoferrin
An antibacterial enzyme originating from acinar cells. Binds iron (iron is used in bacteria replication).

lactoplate test
Measures the amount of **lactoferrin** in the tear film. A non-clinical test.

laevocycloversion
Binocular eye movement in which the upper **corneal** poles of both eyes rotate to the patient's left.

laevoversion
Movement of both eyes to the left.

lagophthalmos
Failure of upper **eyelid** to close completely.

lamellar laceration
A partial-thickness wound of the eye's wall.

lamina
A thin sheet/layer.

lamina cribrosa
A supporting meshwork of **scleral** fibres through which the optic nerve passes.

lamina fusca
The innermost layer of the **sclera**. Contains melanocytes, therefore faintly brown.

Lancaster screen
Similar to a **Hess screen** but uses lines rather than spots of light.

Land's observation
All animals have the same five visuomotor movements.

Landolt C
An **optotype** chart comprising **Sloan letter** Cs, each shown in one of four orientations.

Lang's esopetal factors
Factors that cause a **microtropia** to decompensate.

Lang's two pen test
A gross test of **stereopsis**; the patient attempts to place a pencil on top of another one held by the practitioner.

lantern test
A colour vision test that uses lights. Colours are named, not matched; used for assessing profession suitability.

large metre angle
The combined **binocular** convergence **metre angle.**

LASEK
Acronym of ***laser epithelial keratomileusis.***

LASER
Acronym of light amplification by stimulated emission of radiation.

laser assisted in-situ keratomileusis
A flap is cut in the **corneal stroma** with a **microkeratome**, laser is applied, and the flap is replaced. *Acronym is* ***LASIK.***

laser epithelial keratomileusis
A flap is created with ethanol; laser is applied; the flap is replaced. *Acronym is* ***LASEK.***

lash
Synonym of ***cilia.***

LASIK
Acronym of ***laser assisted in-situ keratomileusis.***

latency
The time from presentation of a stimulus until the start of an electropotential component.

latent hyperopia
Hyperopia in a patient with sufficient accommodative reserves to render themselves emmetropic in most situations.

latent latent nystagmus
Nystagmus that is not present at all until either eye is occluded.

latent nystagmus
Synonym of ***fusion maldevelopment nystagmus syndrome.***

lateral fissure
Divides the frontal and parietal lobes from the temporal lobes.

lateral geniculate body
Synonym of ***lateral geniculate nucleus.***

lateral geniculate nucleus
The part of the visual pathway at which the **optic tract** synapses with the **optic radiations**. Located in the thalamus. *Acronym is **LGN**. Synonym is **lateral geniculate body**.*

lateral inhibition
The ability of a neuron to inhibit the activity of its neighbour(s). Exhibited in the retina in the form of centre-surround **receptive field** organisation. *Synonym is **spatial antagonism**.*

lateral intraparietal area
Brain area involved in movement of the eyes to memorised targets. Projects to the **frontal eye fields** and **superior colliculus**. *Acronym is **LIP**.*

lateral medullary syndrome
Infarction of the lateral medulla oblongata. Clinical symptoms include **Horner's syndrome**, **diplopia**, and torsional **nystagmus**. *Synonym is **Wallenberg syndrome**.*

lateral occipital complex
Brain area involved in grouping of objects using motion cues. *Acronym is **LOC**.*

lateral rectus
L

One of the six **extraocular muscles**. Originates at the **annulus of Zinn** and inserts at the temporal **globe**. Contraction causes **abduction**. Innervated by the **ipsilateral abducens nerve**. *Acronym is **LR**.*

lateropulsion
Describes the situation in which **hypermetric saccades** are made in one direction, and **hypometric saccades** in the other. Classified as either **ipsipulsion** or **contrapulsion**.

lattice degeneration
Peripheral retinal atrophy in a lattice pattern; can cause a **retinal detachment**. Often due to **myopia**. Not to be confused with **lattice dystrophy**.

lattice dystrophy
A **corneal stroma** dystrophy. There are three types (**lattice dystrophy type I**, **lattice dystrophy type II**, and **lattice dystrophy type III**). All are treated by **penetrating keratoplasty**. Not to be confused with **lattice degeneration**.

lattice dystrophy type I
Lattice dystrophy with onset late in the first decade of life with recurrent **corneal erosions**. Fine, spidery branching lines in the **corneal stroma**.

lattice dystrophy type II
Lattice dystrophy with onset in middle age. Similar to **lattice dystrophy type I** but with progressive facial **palsy**. *Synonym is **Meretoja syndrome**.*

lattice dystrophy type III
Lattice dystrophy with onset in the fourth decade of life. Thick ropey lines in the **corneal stroma** with haze.

lazy eye
Synonym of ***amblyopia****.*

LCA
Acronym of ***Leber's congenital amaurosis****/longitudinal chromatic aberration.*

LCD
Acronym of liquid crystal display.

LD
Acronym of learning difficulty.

LDL
Acronym of low density lipoprotein.

LE
Acronym of left eye.

Lea chart
Uses four simple symbols and a matching card to check **visual acuity**. Uses **logMAR** principles.

learning effect
The fact that patients get better at detecting small stimuli after repeated **perimetry** tests.

Leber's congenital amaurosis
No vision at birth. **Oculo-digital sign, nystagmus, relative afferent pupillary defect, hyperopia**. May be associated with **keratoglobus**. *Synonym is* ***early onset macular dystrophy****.*

Leber's hereditary optic neuropathy
Condition occurring between the ages of 15 and 25 years; an X-linked inherited condition. **Disc** redness/swelling, dilated vessels, telangiectatic microangiopathy. *Acronym is* ***LHON****.*

LEE
Acronym of last eye exam.

Lees screen
Instrument for measuring the extent of **strabismus** in different positions of **gaze**, consisting of two panels. The eyes are dissociated by a mirror which causes each eye to view a different screen. Measures up to 30° of eccentric gaze.

lens capsule
The membrane around the lens; this is usually left behind after normal **cataract** surgery. *Synonyms are* ***capsular bag*** *and* ***capsule****.*

lens luxation
Complete dislocation of the lens from the **pupil**. *Synonym is* ***luxation****.*

lens opacity
Synonym of ***cataract***.

lens opacity classification system III
A **cataract** grading scale. *Acronym is* ***LOCS III***.

lens procedure
A refractive surgery in which the lens is replaced.

lens subluxation
Lens luxation when dislocation is partial. Causes multiple refractive errors in one eye. *Synonym is* ***subluxation***.

lensectomy
Removal of the crystalline lens, as performed during **cataract** removal and **refractive lens exchange**.

lenslet
A small lens.

lenticular astigmatism
Astigmatism caused by non-sphericity of the crystalline lens. Any astigmatism not due to **corneal astigmatism** is assumed to be lenticular.

lenticular lens
A lens form adopted for correcting high refractive errors, when providing the full correction over the entire surface of the lens would cause the lens to be exceedingly thick and heavy. The refractive portion of the lens is reduced to a smaller aperture and sits inside a lower-powered carrier lens. This results in a reduced field of view.

lenticular opacity
Synonym of ***cataract***.

lentiglobus
A generalised hemispherical lens deformity.

lentigo maligna
Precancerous **conjunctival melanosis** seen in the elderly, sometimes involving adjacent skin. *Synonym is* ***Hutchinson's freckle***.

leopard fundus
Synonym of ***tesselated fundus***.

LES
Acronym of laser eye surgery.

lesion
Any abnormality of tissue due to disease or trauma.

leucoma
Corneal opacification due to scar tissue. *Synonym is **leukoma**.*

leukaemia
Cancer of the blood or bone marrow.

leukaemic retinopathy
Infiltrates go into the **vitreous humour**, optic nerve, retina, and **choroid**, causing swelling and haze.

leukocoria
A white appearance to the **pupil**. Can be a sign of **retinoblastoma, cataract, Coats' disease, persistent hyperplastic primary vitreous, toxocara** of the **posterior pole, retinopathy of prematurity**, or **retinal detachment**.

leukocytosis
High leukocyte count.

leukoma
*Synonym of **leucoma**.*

levator
*Synonym of **levator palpebrae superioris**.*

levator aponeurosis
Tendon attached to the **levator palpebrae superioris**; divides the two **lacrimal gland** lobes.

levator palpebrae superioris
Muscle that elevates the **tarsus superior**. Innervated by the **caudal central subdivision** via the **oculomotor nerve**. *Synonym is **levator**.*

LG
*Acronym of **lissamine green**.*

LGN
*Acronym of **lateral geniculate nucleus**.*

Lhermitte's hallucinosis
*Synonym of **peduncular hallucinosis**.*

LHON
*Acronym of **Leber's hereditary optic neuropathy**.*

L

lid attached fit
Describes a contact lens which fits with its top held in place by the upper **eyelid**.

lid wiper
The leading edge of the **eyelid** which moves across the **globe** during a blink.

lid wiper epitheliopathy
Lissamine green staining showing damage to the inferior rim of the upper **eyelid** indicates damage to the **lid wiper**; a sign of dry eye syndrome. *Acronym is **LWE**.*

lid-parallel conjunctival folds
Horizontal folds of **conjunctiva** just above the lower **eyelid**, indicative of dry eye syndrome. *Acronym is **LIPCOF**.*

lidocaine
An **amide-linked anaesthetic**, routinely used by **optometrist**s. Typically available at 4% concentration, and with **fluorescein** for **applanation tonometry**. *Synonym is **lignocaine**.*

light adaptation
*Synonym of **adaptation**.*

light stress test
*Synonym of **photostress test**.*

light-near dissociation
Pupils constrict for near, but light response is reduced.

lightness constancy
No matter what the level of background light is, objects appear same relative lightness due to ratio principle.

lignocaine
*Synonym of **lidocaine**.*

lilliputian hallucination
Complex visual **hallucination** in which false, small-scale figures or scenes are perceived. Not the same as **micropsia**, in which real objects appear smaller. Occasionally reported in **Charles Bonnet syndrome**.

limbus
Join between the **cornea** and **sclera/conjunctiva**. A common site of surgical incision.

Lindblom's method
The patient views a horizontal beam of light with both eyes; questions are asked about their perception to ascertain which **extraocular muscle** is **paretic**.

line of Gennari
A white line that extends through the **primary visual cortex** and ends at the border between **V1** and **V2** (hence 'striate' cortex).

LIP
Acronym of ***lateral intraparietal area.***

LIPCOF
Acronym of ***lid-parallel conjunctival folds.***

lipid
Fatty acid + glycerol.

lipid keratopathy
Lipid deposits on the **cornea**. May be **neovascularisation.**

lipid layer
The outermost layer of the tear film. Composed of waxy and cholesterol esters, and polar **lipids**. Polarity prevents evaporation.

lipodermoid
Yellowish-white fatty sub-**conjunctival** dermoid. Slightly larger than **dermoid.**

L

lipofuscin
Orange metabolic product produced by phagocytosis of photoreceptor outer segments and general ageing.

lisch nodules
Small naevi found scattered over the iris; a sign of **neurofibromatosis type 1**.

lissamine green
An alternative to **Rose Bengal stain**; stings less. *Acronym is* ***LG.***

Listing's law
All possible eye positions are reachable by rotation from the **primary position** about **Listing's plane**.

Listing's plane
A single plane in which **Listing's law** states the axes of all eye movements can be found.

lm
Abbreviation of lumens.

LO
Acronym of ***lens opacity.***

LOC
*Acronym of **lateral occipital complex**.*

localisation
Where an object is perceived to be. Compare with **location**.

location
Where an object is in physical space. Compare with **localisation**.

location column
A column perpendicular to surface of cortex in which all cells have the same visual locus. *Synonym is **aggregate field**.*

LOCS III
*Acronym of **lens opacity classification system III**.*

LoG
Acronym of Laplacian of Gaussian operator.

logMAR
A number, representing the logarithm of the minimum angle of resolution. A lower number indicates a better **visual acuity**.

long ciliary nerves
Branch from the nasociliary nerve. Provide sensory innervation to the **globe** and **dilator pupillae**.

long-range motion
Motion that extends beyond a **receptive field**'s spatial and temporal limits. Requires high-level processing. Compare with **short-range motion**.

look optokinetic nystagmus
Optokinetic nystagmus in which the viewer passively views a moving visual scene. Slow phases are longer than in **stare optokinetic nystagmus**.

loop end
Spectacle arm end used for babies – fastened with a ribbon.

loops of Axenfeld
*Synonym of **Axenfeld loops**.*

LOR
Acronym of light output ratio.

loupe
A small magnifying glass-type device, used primarily by surgeons and watchmakers.

low tension glaucoma
*Synonym of **normotensive glaucoma**.*

low vision
Describes any situation in which best-corrected **visual acuity** or **visual fields** are significantly reduced in both eyes. Although there is no specific limit at which a patient is considered to have 'low vision', it should be sufficiently low as to prevent the patient from carrying out certain tasks without the use of **low vision aids**. *Acronym is **LV**. Synonym is **visual impairment**.*

low vision aid
Any device (except spectacles) designed to assist or replace vision for a wide range of tasks. This can include magnifiers, **typoscopes**, talking books, white canes, liquid level indicators, **augmented reality**, and many others. *Acronym is **LVA**.*

LPI
*Acronym of laser **peripheral iridotomy**.*

LPS
Acronym of lipopolysaccharide.

LR
*Acronym of **lateral rectus**.*

LSA
Acronym of longitudinal spherical aberration.

LTF
Acronym of luminous transmission factor.

lucid interval of Vogt
In **senile arcus**, the clear area between the arcus and the **limbus**.

lumen
Unit of **luminous flux**.

luminance
Luminous intensity per area. Typically measured in **candelas** per square metre (units also known as '**nits**'). *Abbreviation is **L**.*

luminance contrast
The difference between luminance of a task and its background.

luminance profile
In one direction across a scene, the changes in luminance expressed as a graph.

luminous efficacy
The ranges of wavelengths from a light source visible to the human eye.

luminous flux
Rate of flow of luminous energy (quantity of light emitted by **source**/received by surface). Measured in **lumens**.

Lundhi loop
*Synonym of **ptosis prop**.*

lutein
A **xanthophyll** found in the **macula**.

lux
Unit of **illuminance**. 1 lux = 1 **lumen**/m².

luxation
*Synonym of **lens luxation**.*

LV
*Acronym of **low vision**.*

LVA
*Acronym of **low vision aid**.*

L

LVC
Acronym of laser vision correction.

LVL
Acronym of low vision leaflet.

LWE
*Acronym of **lid wiper epitheliopathy**.*

Lyme's disease
Autonomic disease caused by **Borrelia** burgdorferi.

lyonisation
The process by which one version of a gene on a female X gene pair is inactivated early in development.

M

M-cells
Abbreviation of ***magno cells.***

M-cone
Abbreviation of green cone.

Ma
Acronym of ***metre angle.***

Mach bands
Visual illusion: a series of grey bars of decreasing luminance, the edges of which are seen as lighter/darker than their neighbour due to the effects of **lateral inhibition.**

machine learning
A set of **artificial intelligence** methods in which a model learns from a training dataset to make decisions about new data. Includes **deep learning.**

macropsia
Perceptual distortion causing objects to appear larger than they are. *Opposite is* ***micropsia.***

M

macula
The central, slightly yellow area of the retina. Contains the **fovea** and **foveola**. *Synonyms are* ***macula lutea*** *and* ***yellow spot.***

macula lutea
Synonym of ***macula.***

macular degeneration
Synonym of ***age-related macular degeneration.***

macular hole
Refers to a lamellar macular hole, macular pseudohole, or **full-thickness macular hole.**

macular pucker
A severe form of **epiretinal membrane.**

macular sparing
The fact that **macula**r vision is often retained when damage occurs to or around the **visual cortex**, due to bilateral projection from each **fovea.**

macular star
Hard exudates streaks centred around the **macula**. Possible causes are **hypertensive retinopathy** and **papilloedema.**

macular translocation
Surgical procedure in which the **macula** is moved to another location.

maculopathy
Any **macular** pathology.

madarosis
Loss of **eyelash**es or eyebrows (non-manually).

Maddox double prism test
Two equal prisms with fused bases are presented in front of one eye to induce **monocular** diplopia. In a state of **orthophoria**, the fellow eye should see an image directly in the middle of the **diplopic** images. Prism can be introduced to reach this state.

Maddox rod
A trial set lens with no refractive power but a series of parallel grooves that reduce form perception and cause light to appear as streaks. Introduced in front of one eye and used to determine dissociated deviation of the eyes.

Maddox wing
A device used to measure near dissociated deviation of the eyes. It consists of two sets of numbers (one for vertical deviations and one for horizontal), and a septum, which dissociates the eyes. On the opposing side of the septum are arrows which are used to indicate the amount of deviation present.

M

magnetic resonance imaging
Neuroimaging technique that measures changes in the spin of hydrogen atoms induced by transient changes in a magnetic field. *Acronym is* ***MRI****.*

magnetic resonance spectroscopy
Magnetic resonance imaging technique that estimates localised metabolite concentrations in tissue. *Synonym is* ***chemical shift imaging****.*

magneto-optical effects
A number of phenomena seen when an electromagnetic wave propagates through a magnetic field.

magno cells
Cells that form part of the **magnocellular pathway**. *Abbreviation is* ***M-cells****. Synonym is* ***phasic cells****.*

magnocellular pathway
Sub-pathway of the visual system that contains info about flicker, movement, location, and low-**contrast** stimuli. Achromatic. Poor resolution.

main sequence of saccades
Term used to describe the correlation between amplitude, duration, and velocity of **saccade**s.

major amblyoscope
Any **amblyoscope** mounted to a table.

make-up spectacles
Spectacles with lenses that flip out of the way so the patient can put in contact lenses or apply make-up to one eye at a time.

malattia leventinese
Synonym of ***dominant drusen.***

Mallett unit
Device used to measure **associated phoria**. Composed of four **Nonius lines** and a binocular **fusion** locking element. A **distance Mallett unit** and **near Mallett unit** is available.

MALT
Acronym of ***mucosa-associated lymphoid tissue.***

Mandelbaum effect
The tendency of the eye to **accommodate** at near in conditions of poor visibility.

manifest latent nystagmus
Latent nystagmus that is always present due to some sort of **fusion**-preventing ocular abnormality (e.g. **cataract, strabismus**, etc.) but which gets worse when either eye is occluded.

M

MAO
Acronym of monoamine oxidase.

MAOI
Acronym of monoamine oxidase inhibitor.

map-dot-fingerprint dystrophy
Synonym of ***Cogan's microcystic dystrophy.***

MAR
Acronym of minimum angle of resolution/multi anti-reflective coat.

Marcus Gunn jaw winking
Synonym of ***jaw winking.***

Marcus Gunn pupil
Synonym of ***relative afferent pupillary defect.***

Marcus Gunn test
Synonym of ***swinging flashlight test.***

Marfan syndrome
Elastic fibre disorder. Causes long limbs and fingers, crowded teeth, and **myopia**. Can cause **ectopia lentis**, **retinal detachment**, and **glaucoma**.

marginal orbicularis
Most central portion of the **orbicularis oculi**.

marginal tissue
Tissue that separates the optic nerve from the **choroid** and **sclera**. *Synonym is **border tissue**.*

Margolis eye throwing technique
Rehabilitative technique for **unilateral neglect**, in which patients are encouraged to make large saccades into their neglected field.

Marie–Strümpell disease
*Synonym of **ankylosing spondylitis**.*

Marinesco–Sjögren syndrome
Rare congenital disorder that includes congenital **cataract** as a sign.

Marr and Nishihara object recognition model
Theory of object recognition that states that all 3D shapes are broken into **generalised cones**. This theory allows for **viewpoint invariance**.

Marr–Hildreth computational model
Mathematical method for edge detection in image analysis. The image is Gaussian smoothed, and the Laplacian operator of the two-dimensional luminance profile provides the location of edges.

Martegiani funnel
Area at the top of the **optic disc** that marks the beginning of the **hyaloid canal**.

maxilla
The bone of the upper jaw.

Maxwell's spot
Entoptic phenomenon: a central dark red spot seen when observing a purple light. Occurs because the **macula** contains blue-absorbing **carotenoid**s, making the central **visual field** appear darker.

McGurk effect
The fact that vision and sound are combined to form a percept, sometimes misleadingly.

MCOT
Acronym of minimum critical oxygen tension.

MCT
Acronym of modified clinical technique.

MD
Acronym of ***mean deviation.***

MDP
Acronym of motion detection perimetry.

mean deviation
On a **perimetry** printout, the mean difference in threshold as compared to age-normative data across the whole **visual field**, indicating global changes in sensitivity. *Acronym is MD.*

mean sphere
The overall average power of a lens, ignoring cylindrical power. Calculated by adding half the cylindrical power to the sphere power.

Meares–Irlen syndrome
Synonym of ***visual stress.***

media opacity
Any opacity within the eye.

medial longitudinal fasciculus
Interneuron bundle that connects the **oculomotor nerve**, **trochlear nerve**, and **abducens nerve** together. *Acronym is MLF.*

medial rectus
One of the six **extraocular muscle**s. Originates at the **annulus of Zinn** and inserts at the nasal **globe**. Contraction causes **adduction**. Innervated by the **ipsilateral oculomotor nerve**.

medial vestibular nucleus
In the pons, receives input from the **semicircular canal**s of the inner ear. Transmits via the **oculomotor nerve**. *Acronym is MVN.*

medulloepithelioma
Rare embryonic **uveal** tumour, usually of the **ciliary body**. Described as 'teratoid' or 'non-teratoid'. *Synonym is* ***diktyoma.***

Meesmann dystrophy
An anterior **corneal** dystrophy presenting in patients under 10 years of age with mild visual symptoms. Looks like raindrops on a window.

MEG
Acronym of magnetoencephalography.

megalocornea
Enlargement of the **cornea** (more than 13 mm diameter), without loss of clarity.

megalopapilla
Large **optic disc**.

meibomian gland
Sebaceous glands located posterior to **lashes** on upper and lower **eyelids**. Produce the **meibum** of the **lipid layer** of the tear film. *Synonym is **tarsal gland**.*

meibomian gland dysfunction
Common condition in which **meibum** composition is altered, leading to keratinisation of the **meibomian gland** walls. The ducts become blocked, and meibum changes from clear to opaque. Reduction in the **lipid layer** of the tear film causes tears to evaporate more readily, leading to symptoms of dryness. *Acronym is **MGD**.*

meibomian gland granuloma
*Synonym of **chalazion**.*

meibomian oil
*Synonym of **meibum**.*

M

meibum
Produced by the **meibomian glands**; forms a major component of the **lipid layer** of the tear film. Comprises lipids and proteins. *Synonym is **meibomian oil**.*

melanocytoma
Asymptomatic unilateral congenital **choroidal** **lesion**. Large, black, at inferior **disc**.

melanocytosis
*Synonym of **melanosis**.*

melanoma
Cancer of melanocytes. Can be found in the eye, usually in the **choroid**.

melanosis
Hyperpigmentation due to **hypertrophy** or **hyperplasia** of melanocytes. *Synonym is **melanocytosis**.*

melanosis oculi
*Synonym of **subepithelial melanosis**.*

melanosome
Present in the skin and **retinal pigment epithelium** (greatest concentration behind the **fovea**). Produced until 2 years old.

MEM
*Acronym of **monocular estimation method**.*

meninges
Membranes that cover the brain and spinal cord. From inner to outer, the **pia mater, arachnoid**, and **dura mater**. *Singular is **meninx**.*

meningioma
Cancer of the **meninges**.

meninx
*Singular of **meninges**.*

Meretoja syndrome
*Synonym of **lattice dystrophy type II**.*

meridional amblyopia
Amblyopia causing reduced sensitivity to stimuli with a specific orientation, usually due to high **astigmatism**. *Synonym is **astigmatic amblyopia**.*

Merkel cell carcinoma
Rare, highly malignant tumour. Red/purple. More common in elderly women.

mesencephalic reticular formation
Found adjacent to the nucleus of the **oculomotor nerve**. The **gaze** control centre of the brain for **vergence**. Contains the **rostral interstitial nucleus of the medial longitudinal fasciculus** and the **interstitial nucleus of Cajal**. *Acronym is MRF.*

meso-zeaxanthin
A **xanthophyll** found in the **macula**.

mesopic
Mid-range **illumination** levels in which both rods and cones are responsive.

metamorphopsia
Objects appear distorted in shape, size, and **location**, due to, for example, raised **macula**/intoxication/**migraine**/neurosis.

method of adjustment
One of the **classical psychophysical methods** of threshold estimation in which stimulus intensity is altered by the test subject until it is first perceived or not perceived.

method of constant stimuli
One of the **classical psychophysical methods** in which stimuli are presented at a variety of fixed intensities in a random order, multiple times. A **psychometric function** is constructed from the number of times each stimulus is perceived, and threshold is estimated, usually at the intensity at which the stimulus was perceived on 75% of presentations.

M

method of limits
One of the **classical psychophysical methods** of threshold estimation in which stimulus intensity is altered in regular steps until it is first perceived or not perceived.

metre angle
Measurement unit of **convergence**. Reciprocal of **fixation** distance. Does not account for **interpupillary distance**. *Acronym is* ***Ma***.

Meyer's loop
The portion of the **optic radiations** that pass around the temporal lobe (inferior retina/superior field).

MFS
Acronym of ***Miller Fisher syndrome***.

MGD
Acronym of ***meibomian gland dysfunction***.

MHC
Acronym of major histocompatibility complex.

MI
Acronym of myocardial infarction.

M

Michelson contrast
Contrast defined as the variation in luminance within a visual scene, divided by double the mean luminance.

microaneurysm
A tiny **aneurysm**.

microbial infiltrative keratitis
Painful **cornea**l infection with epithelial defects, severe corneal suppuration, **uveitis**, and central **lesions** >1 mm in size. *Acronym is* ***MIK***. *Synonyms are* ***infectious keratitis, microbial keratitis, suppurative keratitis****, and* ***ulcerative keratitis***.

microbial keratitis
Synonym of ***microbial infiltrative keratitis***.

microkeratome
Small surgical instrument used to make a **cornea**l flap in laser surgery.

microphakia
Abnormally small crystalline lens diameter. Can be associated with Lowe's syndrome.

microphthalmia
Synonym of ***microphthalmos***.

microphthalmos
Congenital condition in which the eyes are abnormally small. *Synonym is **microphthalmia**.*

micropsia
Perceptual distortion causing objects to appear smaller than they are. May be due to elevation of the **macula** or of neurological origin. *Opposite is **macropsia**.*

microsaccade
Constant eye movements in apparently random directions. Improve perception of fine spatial detail and prevent fading of the retinal image via the **Troxler effect**.

microspherophakia
Microphakia with a spherical lens shape.

microsporidal keratitis
Opportunistic bacterial infection of the **cornea**.

microtropia
A small angle **strabismus** (usually <10 Δ) in which some form of binocular single vision occurs.

microtropia with identity
Microtropia in which the patient exhibits **eccentric fixation** and no movement on cover test. **Harmonious anomalous retinal correspondence** is present.

microtropia without identity
Microtropia in which there is a small movement found on cover test. Patient can have **abnormal retinal correspondence** or normal **retinal correspondence** with central **suppression** and peripheral **fusion**.

midget cells
*Synonym of **parvo cells**.*

migraine
Two types: **common migraine** and **classic migraine**.

migraine aura
Visual symptoms that can precede or accompany a **classic migraine**. May occur in isolation (**acephalgic migraine**). Including, but not limited to: positive/negative **scotomas**, scintillating scotoma, **chromatophenes**, **teichopsia**, and transient **visual field** loss.

migraine sine migraine
*Synonym of **acephalgic migraine**.*

MIK
*Acronym of **microbial infiltrative keratitis**.*

M

milia
Painless white papules sometimes found around the eyes that tend to appear in clusters.

Mill's balance
An instrument with similar design to a **Maddox wing** but with separate charts for measuring vertical and horizontal deviation, and with smaller text (providing a better stimulus for **accommodation**).

Miller Fisher syndrome
A rare cause of ophthalmoplegia. A form of Guillain–Barré syndrome. *Acronym is **MFS**. Synonym is **Fisher syndrome**.*

mini bevel
A lens edge bevel with a 'shoulder'. Used in high powered negative lenses to reduce the power ring effect. *Synonym is **easy V**.*

minimum amplitude zone
Similar to a **null zone** but refers to the position of **gaze** that causes the greatest reduction specifically in **nystagmus amplitude** rather than **nystagmus intensity**.

minus lens
A concave lens.

miosis
Pupil constriction.

miotic
Any chemical that can cause **miosis**.

mixed astigmatism
Astigmatism in which the foci lines lie either side of the retina.

mixed reality
*Synonym of **augmented reality**.*

mkd
Abbreviation of marked deviation.

MLF
*Acronym of **medial longitudinal fasciculus**.*

Möbius syndrome
Condition in which the abducens and facial nerves fail to develop. Causes developmental delay, deafness, **lagophthalmos**, and a horizontal **gaze** weakness.

mod
Abbreviation of moderate deviation.

modified logMAR
1–**logMAR** score. Used to make higher scores sound better to the patient.

modified monovision
Using **multifocal contact lens**es but having one with more of an emphasis on near vision and one with an emphasis on distance.

modified Nott retinoscopy
Fixation target is placed at the child's working distance; the practitioner moves 0.75 D behind the target. A 'with' movement of the **retinoscopy** reflex indicates the patient has **accommodative lag**.

modified OXO test
The test for **harmonious anomalous retinal correspondence/suppression** found on a **near Mallett unit**.

modified Thorington test
An alternative to the **Maddox rod** test for measuring **heterophoria** (as a spotlight alone is a poor accommodative target). A torch is shone through a **Thorington card**, whilst a Maddox rod is held in front of one eye. The patient is instructed first to view the card, followed by the line formed by the light through the Maddox rod. The position of the line on the Thorington card indicates the size of the **phoria**.

modulus of elasticity
A surface's tendency to be deformed elastically (non-permanently) when force is applied. A characteristic applicable to contact lenses. *Opposite is* ***modulus of rigidity****. Synonym is* ***Young's modulus****.*

modulus of rigidity
Opposite of ***modulus of elasticity****.*

MOE
Acronym of mean oblique error.

Moh's surgery
Highly effective method of removing a **basal cell carcinoma** – the **carcinoma** is removed, and the **marginal tissue** around the excised **lesion** is tested histologically – if this tissue is found to be cancerous, more tissue is removed until non-cancerous tissue is found at the surgical margins.

Mohindra technique
Performing **retinoscopy** at near (50 cm), in the dark with one of the patient's eyes occluded.

Moll glands
Sweat glands of the **eyelid**s. Located anterior to the **tarsal plates**.

M

molluscum contagiosum
Viral infection causing follicular **conjunctivitis** and wart-like growths on the ocular **adnexa**. Found in AIDS. Treated by excavation.

Molteno implant
Device placed half-inside the eye, which drains **aqueous humour** (used if **trabeculectomy** closes itself). *Synonym is **Molteno shunt**.*

Molteno shunt
*Synonym of **Molteno implant**.*

monocular
One eye.

monocular estimation method
Dynamic retinoscopy performed with a near target and **retinoscope** at a fixed distance. Briefly introduce spherical lenses to measure **accommodative lag** or **accommodative lead**. *Acronym is MEM.*

monocular temporal crescent
The portion of the binocular **visual field** seen by one eye only. Approximately 30° per eye.

M

monophasic square-wave intrusion
A type of **square-wave intrusion** commonly seen in normal patients. After fixating for a short time, a horizontal **saccade** moves the eyes off **fixation**, followed by a short gap and a corrective saccade.

monovision
Situation in which one eye is used for near vision and the other for distance.

moon illusion
Visual illusion in which the moon, when near the horizon, appears larger than it does when higher in the sky. Partially explained by **equidistance tendency**.

Moore's lightning streaks
Vertical white **photopsia** seen in **scotopic** conditions. Indicates **posterior vitreous detachment**.

Mooren's ulcer
Ulceration of the **cornea**. Begins in periphery and spreads centrally. Painful. May involve **sclera**.

MOP
Acronym of mean oblique power.

Morgagnian cataract
A hypermature **cataract** that has been autolysed.

morning glory
Severe **coloboma** of the **optic disc** (much larger than an **optic disc pit**). 'Sunrise' appearance of the optic disc. Poor visual function.

mosaic dominance
The case in binocular vision in which parts of a (large) stimulus are ignored in favour of another stimulus seen by the fellow eye.

mosaic fundus
Synonym of ***tesselated fundus.***

mosaic rivalry
In binocular vision, when two completely unfuseable stimuli are seen by each eye, random segments of each are seen at different times.

motility
Synonym of ***ocular motility.***

motility test
Clinical test to detect **incomitance** and measure accuracy of **smooth pursuit**. The patient is asked to follow a target whilst the **corneal reflex**es are observed.

motion after effect
Motion-specific **receptive field**s can fatigue, altering motion perception. This is a **cortical** process (occurring in the **visual cortex** and **visual area middle temporal**).

motion blindness
Synonym of ***akinetopsia.***

motion coherence threshold
The signal-to-noise ratio required to make judgements about the movement of moving stimuli.

motor fusion
The ability to maintain sensory **fusion** through a range of **vergence** movements.

mouches volantes
Synonym of ***muscae volitantes.***

MR
Acronym of ***Maddox rod/medial rectus.***

MRF
Acronym of ***mesencephalic reticular formation.***

MRI
Acronym of ***magnetic resonance imaging.***

mRNA
Acronym of messenger ribonucleic acid.

MS
Acronym of ***mean sphere****/multiple sclerosis.*

MST
Acronym of ***visual area medial superior temporal****.*

MT
Acronym of ***visual area middle temporal****.*

mucin balls
Deposits sometimes found under contact lenses.

mucosa-associated lymphoid tissue
Concentrated regions of lymphoid tissue found in the body. One such region is in the **conjunctiva (conjunctival-associated lymphoid tissue)**. *Acronym is* ***MALT****.*

mucous layer
The base layer of the tear film containing large **glycoproteins**, **glycosaminoglycans**, etc. Hydrophilic. Maintains tear film stability during blinks.

M

Müller cells
Glial cells in the retina. Run from the **inner limiting membrane** to the **outer limiting membrane**.

Müller-Lyer illusion
Visual illusion of two lines of the same length with oppositely pointing arrowheads. Due to perspective cues, the line with the inwardly pointing arrowheads appears to be larger.

Müller's muscles
Help in maintaining palpebral aperture. *Synonym is* ***tarsal muscles****.*

multifocal contact lens
A type of **simultaneous vision contact lens** with an aspheric power change giving both distance and near portions.

Munsell colour system
An old system of defining colours; comprising 40 hues at different 'values' of brightness and different 'chromas' of saturation.

Munsell tree
3D way of representing the **Munsell colour system**.

Munson's sign
V-shape in lower **eyelid** when looking down. Indicative of **corneal ectasia**.

muscae volitantes
Floaters when caused by embryological debris. *Synonym is **mouches volantes**.*

muscle sequelae
Sequence of changes observed in **extraocular muscle** function following paralytic **strabismus** of a muscle. Following the initial palsy, the **contralateral synergist** becomes overactive. Next, there is overaction of the **ipsilateral antagonist**, and finally the **contralateral** antagonist exhibits a secondary underaction. *Synonym is **sequelae**.*

mutton fat keratic precipitates
Keratic precipitates with a large, greasy appearance. Sign of granulomatous disease.

MVN
*Acronym of **medial vestibular nucleus**.*

MW
Acronym of molecular weight.

myalgia
Muscle pain.

myasthenia gravis
Neuromuscular weakness. Skeletal muscle weaker during activity, better at rest. Causes **ptosis**.

mydriasis
Dilation of the **pupil**. *Synonyms are **dilatation** and **dilation**.*

mydriatic
Any chemical that can cause **mydriasis**.

myelinated nerve fibres
Condition in which myelination of the optic nerve continued after birth. White appearance to the area around the **optic nerve head**. Not usually a problem unless the **macula** is involved.

myoclonus
Muscle spasms.

myodesopsia
Perception of **floaters**.

myogenic
*Synonym of **myopathy**.*

myokymia
Twitch of muscle when there is no weakness.

myopathy
A form of **paresis** or paralysis due to muscle **lesion**. *Synonym is **myogenic**.*

myope
An individual with **myopia**.

myopia
Condition in which parallel light is focused in front of the retina when **accommodation** is relaxed. *Synonyms are **nearsighted** and **nearsightedness**.*

myopic crescent
Patchy area on temporal **optic disc** margin, suggests **myopia**. *Synonym is **temporal crescent**.*

myotonic dystrophy
Patients have **ptosis**, an expressionless face, frontal balding, **Christmas tree cataract**s. Often have diabetes mellitus.

N

NAD
Acronym of no abnormality detected/no apparent defect/not actually done.

naevus
Lesion containing naevocytes which in turn contain **melanosomes**, which create melanin. A **benign tumour**.

naevus of Ota
Synonym of ***oculodermal melanosis.***

NaFl
Abbreviation of ***sodium fluorescein.***

nagel
A type of **anomaloscope**.

NAION
Acronym of ***non-arteritic anterior ischaemic optic neuropathy.***

nanophthalmos
Microphthalmos when there is nothing else wrong.

nasal retinal disparity
Synonym of ***uncrossed retinal disparity.***

nasal step
Synonym of ***Rønne nasal step.***

nasalisation
Central retinal vessel trunk leans nasally in a cup with significant **glaucoma**tous nerve loss.

nasion
Part of the skull at bridge of nose – used as a reference point when attaching electrodes.

naso-temporal optokinetic asymmetry
The fact that, in early visual development, **optokinetic nystagmus** only responds to horizontal stimuli moving in the nasalward direction for each eye. This asymmetry is preserved in adults with **fusion maldevelopment nystagmus syndrome**.

nasociliary nerve
A branch of the ophthalmic nerve. Branches into, amongst others, the long ciliary nerves.

nasolacrimal duct
Carries tears from the **lacrimal sac** to the nose. *Acronym is **NLD**. Synonym is **tear duct**.*

nasvacometer
A circular nomogram tool used to convert between **Snellen fraction** required to see an object and the distance from and size of that object.

NATTD
*Acronym of **nightblindness-associated transient tonic downgaze**.*

NCT
Acronym of non-contact tonometry.

ND
Acronym of neutral density.

near esotropia
An **esotropia** that is manifest at near viewing.

near exotropia
An **exotropia** that is manifest at near viewing.

near Mallett unit
A **Mallett unit** for use at the patient's habitual reading distance. *Acronym is **nMU**.*

near point of accommodation
The closest distance that an individual can focus using the full extent of their accommodative reserves. *Acronym is **NPA**. Synonym is **punctum proximum**.*

near point of convergence
The closest distance that an individual can converge the eyes to. *Acronym is **NPC**.*

near synkinesis
*Synonym of **near vision triad**.*

near vision effectivity error
The fact that the form of lenses and gaps between lenses used in a subjective **refraction** cause a slight error in the calculation of a patient's reading prescription.

near vision triad
Collective term for the **accommodation**, **convergence**, and **miosis** that occur when fixating a near object. *Synonym is **near synkinesis**.*

nearsighted
*Synonym of **myopia**.*

nearsightedness
Synonym of ***myopia****.*

nedocromil
An anti-inflammatory mast cell stabiliser.

NEG
Acronym of non-enzymatic glycation.

negative fusional reserve
The **fusional reserve** measured using base in prism. *Synonym is* ***divergence fusional reserve****.*

negative fusional vergence
The **fusional vergence** limit in response to base in prism. *Acronym is* ***NFV****.*

negative relative accommodation
The amount of positive spherical power that can be added to an initial reading **addition** before blurring or **diplopia** is experienced by the patient. *Acronym is* ***NRA****.*

negative retinal disparity
Synonym of ***uncrossed retinal disparity****.*

negative scotoma
A **scotoma** that is not perceived as a 'hole' in the vision but which is 'filled in' by the brain. The physiological blind spot is an example of this.

neophyte
A beginner. Often used to describe first-time contact lens or spectacle wearers.

neoplasm
Tumour.

neovascular age-related macular degeneration
Synonym of ***wet age-related macular degeneration****.*

neovascular glaucoma
Glaucoma caused by reduction in aqueous outflow through the **trabecular meshwork** due to **neovascularisation** of the **anterior chamber angle**.

neovascularisation
Growth of new blood vessels.

nerve fibre layer
Composed of **gangliocyte** axons and astrocytes. *Acronym is* ***NFL****.*

neural aniseikonia
Perceived difference in retinal image size, due to unusual retinal element layout.

neural integrator
Part(s) of the brain involved in maintaining **gaze** by **tonic innervation**: the **nucleus prepositus hypoglossi** (for horizontal gaze holding) and the **interstitial nucleus of Cajal** (vertical and torsional gaze).

neural net
*Synonym of **neural network**.*

neural network
In **deep learning**, a set of interconnected nodes arranged in layers, each of which transform data from previous nodes. *Synonyms are **artificial neural network** and **neural net**.*

neuralgia
Pain experienced due to damage or disease of a nerve.

neurofibromatosis type 1
Hereditary condition causing **Lisch nodules** and **ectropion uveae**. Often associated with optic nerve **glioma**. *Acronym is **NF-1**. Synonym is **von Recklinghausen disease**.*

neuroretinitis
Inflammation of both the retina and **optic nerve head**.

neutral density filter bar
Used to determine how much of a reduction in **illuminance** is tolerated by an eye before **suppression** occurs.

new vessels elsewhere
Describes leaking vessels >1 **disc diameter** from the **optic disc**; found in **diabetic retinopathy**.

NF-1
*Acronym of **neurofibromatosis type 1**.*

NFL
*Acronym of **nerve fibre layer**.*

NFV
*Acronym of **negative fusional vergence**.*

NIBUT
Acronym of non-invasive tear breakup time.

NIDD
Acronym of non-insulin-dependent diabetes.

night myopia
Tonic accommodation occurring when it is not completely dark. Frequently manifests during night driving. Patients may benefit from −0.50 overcorrection in these situations.

nightblindness
*Synonym of **nyctalopia**.*

nightblindness-associated transient tonic downgaze
Infant boys with **congenital stationary nightblindness** may exhibit a chin-up **abnormal head posture** with the eyes tonically in downgaze, with high-frequency low-amplitude horizontal pendular **nystagmus**. *Acronym is **NATTD**.*

nipping
The effect of high arterial pressure causing an underlying vein to be compressed at the site of the crossing. A sign seen in **hypertensive retinopathy**. *Synonym is **Gunn's sign**.*

nit
Occasionally used to refer to **candela**s per square metre (unit of **luminance**).

NITBUT
Acronym of non-invasive tear breakup time.

NK cell
Abbreviation of natural killer cell.

NLD
*Acronym of **nasolacrimal duct**.*

nMU
*Acronym of **near Mallett unit**.*

nodular drusen
*Synonym of **hard drusen**.*

non-arteritic anterior ischaemic optic neuropathy
Occurs in patients between 45 and 65 years of age. **Pallor** and **oedema** of the **optic disc**, few splinter haemorrhages and hyperfluorescent **fundus fluorescein angiography**. Often occurs on waking. *Acronym is **NAION**.*

non-contact tonometer
Any type of **tonometer** that does not make physical contact with the patient's eye.

non-exudative age-related macular degeneration
*Synonym of **dry age-related macular degeneration**.*

non-ischaemic retinal vein occlusion
Causes reduction in **visual acuity, optic disc** oedema, **macular** oedema, **cotton wool spots, dot haemorrhages, blot haemorrhages, flame haemorrhages, relative afferent pupillary defect**.

N

non-proliferative sickle cell retinopathy
Causes **salmon patches**, **black sunbursts**, and retinal holes.

Nonius line
One of the four red lines that are viewed monocularly on a Mallett unit.

normal
In optics, the line perpendicular to a refractive/reflective surface.

normal tension glaucoma
*Synonym of **normotensive glaucoma**.*

normotensive glaucoma
Glaucoma in which **intraocular pressure** is within the normally acceptable limits. This type of glaucoma accounts for ⅓ of all glaucoma patients, and it is more often elderly patients. Splinter haemorrhages at the **disc** are a sign. *Acronym is NTG. Synonyms are **low tension glaucoma** and **normal tension glaucoma**.*

North Carolina macular dystrophy
Rare inherited condition that presents in 1st–2nd decades of life. Causes **drusen** and atrophy at the **macula**.

NOT
Acronym of nucleus of the optic tract.

N

Nott retinoscopy
Dynamic retinoscopy in which the distance of the **retinoscope** is adjusted. **Accommodative lag** or **accommodative lead** is the dioptric distance between the retinoscope and the target at the point of neutrality.

novelty preference
Method of checking **visual acuity** in babies – they will instinctively look towards new things they can see.

NPA
*Acronym of **near point of accommodation**.*

NPC
*Acronym of **near point of convergence**.*

NPH
*Acronym of **nucleus prepositus hypoglossi**.*

NPL
Acronym of no perception of light.

NRA
Acronym of ***negative relative accommodation.***

NRC
Acronym of normal retinal correspondence.

NS
Acronym of ***nuclear sclerosis.***

NSAID
Acronym of non-steroidal anti-inflammatory drug.

NTG
Acronym of ***normotensive glaucoma.***

nuclear cataract
Synonym of ***nuclear sclerosis.***

nuclear sclerosis
Common form of **brunescent cataract** caused usually by ageing. Causes **myopia;** may lead to **angle closure glaucoma.** *Acronym is NS. Synonym is* ***nuclear cataract.***

nucleus prepositus hypoglossi
The **neural integrator** for horizontal eye movements. *Acronym is NPH.*

null point
Synonym of ***null zone.***

null position
Synonym of ***null zone.***

null zone
The position(s) of **gaze** which cause **nystagmus intensity** to be at a minimum. Not to be confused with the **minimum amplitude zone**. *Synonyms are* ***null point*** *and* ***null position.***

nummular
Coin-shaped.

NV
*Acronym of near vision/****neovascularisation.***

NVA
Acronym of neovascularisation of the anterior chamber angle.

nvCJD
Acronym of new variant Creutzfeldt–Jakob disease.

N

NVD
Acronym of neovascularisation of the optic disc.

NVE
Acronym of neovascularisation elsewhere.

NVI
Acronym of neovascularisation of the iris.

NVP
Acronym of near vision point.

NWT
Acronym of normal wearing time.

nyctalopia
Nightblindness. Occasionally (incorrectly) referred to as **hemeralopia**. *Synonym is* ***nightblindness***.

nystagmat
An individual with **nystagmus.**

nystagmus
Regular, repetitive movement of the eyes containing (at least) a slow (drifting) phase. Can be induced physiologically, may be **acquired nystagmus** or **infantile onset nystagmus**.

nystagmus amplitude
The total size of ocular oscillation seen in a patient with **nystagmus**.

nystagmus block syndrome
Esotropia that develops to compensate for **nystagmus**. In this condition, **nystagmus amplitude** is greatest in the **primary position**. There is no **dissociated vertical deviation**. *Synonym is* ***nystagmus compensation syndrome***.

nystagmus compensation syndrome
Synonym of ***nystagmus block syndrome***.

nystagmus frequency
The frequency with which the eyes oscillate in a patient with **nystagmus**. Recorded in Hz.

nystagmus intensity
A value calculated by multiplying **nystagmus amplitude** by **nystagmus frequency**.

nystagmus waveform
The characteristic pattern of oscillations seen in a patient with **nystagmus**. Many different waveforms can occur, even in the same patient.

O

OAG
Acronym of ***open angle glaucoma.***

OBF
Acronym of ocular blood flow.

object-centred unilateral neglect
Unilateral neglect of one half of individual objects.

objective fronto-parallel plane
The physical plane in front of and parallel to the eyes.

oblate
Describes a curve that steepens in the periphery.

oblique astigmatism
Astigmatism in which the negative cylindrical power's **axis** is more than 15° either side of 180 or 90.

OC
Acronym of ***optical centre.***

occipital cortex
Synonym of ***visual cortex.***

occipital lobe
The lobe of the brain containing the **visual cortex**. *Synonym is* ***visual lobe.***

occlusion amblyopia
Amblyopia due to **iatrogenic** over-patching.

occult choroidal neovascularisation
Choroidal neovascularisation in which the **choroidal neovascular membrane** is below the **retinal pigment epithelium** and so shows up poorly on **fluorescein angiography**. Has a better prognosis because the **neovascularisation** is limited by retinal pigment epithelium.

ochre membrane
A yellow appearance to the **vitreous humour** due to compacted blood, due to **intragel haemorrhage**.

OCR
Acronym of ***optical character recognition.***

ocriplasmin
Intravitreal injection that aims to break down vitreoretinal attachments in cases of **idiopathic full-thickness macular hole**.

OCT
Acronym of ***optical coherence tomography.***

ocular albinism
Form of **albinism** presenting primarily in the eyes, as opposed to **oculocutaneous albinism**. On examination there is a red, transilluminative appearance to the irides and hypopigmented retinas.

ocular apraxia
Synonym of ***saccade initiation failure.***

ocular fibrillation
Synonym of ***voluntary nystagmus.***

ocular flutter
A saccadic abnormality in which rapid back-to-back horizontal **saccade**s occur.

ocular histoplasmosis
Synonym of ***presumed ocular histoplasmosis syndrome.***

ocular hypertension
An eye with high **intraocular pressure** – usually defined as >21 mmHg but without any other signs of **glaucoma**. *Acronym is* ***OHT.***

ocular melanocytosis
Synonym of ***subepithelial melanosis.***

ocular migraine
Migraine originating at the retina. Causes **scotoma**, and may cause headache. *Synonym is* ***retinal migraine.***

ocular motility
The state of binocular **comitance**. Investigated with the **motility test**. *Acronym is* ***OM.*** *Synonym is* ***motility.***

ocular pemphigoid
Conjunctivitis, **hyperaemia**, mucus, vesicles which burst, leaving ulcers. May lead to **symblepharon** or **ankyloblepharon**.

Ocular Response Analyser
A **non-contact tonometer** that also measures **central corneal thickness**; **corneal hysteresis**, and **corneal** resistance factor.

ocular shuddering
Synonym of ***voluntary nystagmus.***

ocular straylight
Glare caused by the eye (e.g. due to media opacity, hypopigmentation, etc.).

ocular thermography
Investigative technique, examining the temperature of the front of the eye, primarily to assess the tear film.

ocular torticollis
Synonym of ***abnormal head posture.***

ocularist
Someone who designs and makes prosthetic eyes.

oculist
Outdated term that previously referred to an **ophthalmologist** or **optometrist**.

oculo-digital sign
Phenomenon in which blind children may rub their eyes to stimulate flashes of light. This may, if done excessively, cause **enophthalmos**. *Synonym is* ***Franceschetti's oculo-digital sign.***

oculocephalic reflex
Vestibulo-ocular reflex in response to turning the head. Usually performed on an unconscious patient to assess brain function. *Synonym is* ***doll's eye reflex.***

oculocutaneous albinism
Similar to **ocular albinism**, but the skin is hypopigmented as well. Diagnosis is enhanced by the **tyrosinase hair bulb test**.

oculodermal melanosis
A hyperpigmentation commonly seen on the **conjunctiva** and skin around the eyes. *Synonyms are* ***naevus of Ota*** *and* ***Ota's naevus.***

oculography
The recording of eye position and movement.

oculometer
Any device used to track movement of the **eyeballs**.

oculomotor apraxia
Synonym of ***saccade initiation failure.***

O

oculomotor nerve
Cranial nerve III. Innervates the **ipsilateral medial rectus, inferior rectus, inferior oblique, levator palpebrae superioris** and **ciliary ganglion**, and the **contralateral superior rectus.** *Synonym is **third cranial nerve**.*

oculomotor range
The 'normal' range of eye movements: ~80° horizontally and ~60° vertically.

oculopalatal myoclonus
*Synonym of **oculopalatal tremor**.*

oculopalatal tremor
A primarily horizontal **acquired nystagmus** in which the eye movements are synchronous with movements of the palate. *Synonym is **oculopalatal myoclonus**.*

oculotonic crisis
Eyes tonically fixed in **elevation** bilaterally, usually as a reaction to medication.

oculus dexter
Right eye (Latin).

oculus sinister
Left eye (Latin). *Acronym is **OS**.*

oculus unitas
*Synonym of **oculus utro**.*

oculus uniter
*Synonym of **oculus utro**.*

oculus uterque
*Synonym of **oculus utro**.*

oculus utro
Both eyes (Latin). *Acronym is **OU**. Synonyms are **oculus unitas**, **oculus uniter**, and **oculus uterque**.*

OD
*Acronym of **oculus dexter**/optical centre for distance/to be taken once daily.*

oedema
Swelling caused by accumulation of fluid.

offset cylinder technique
When performing the **Jackson cross cylinder** test, the practice of deliberately misaligning the cylinder **axis** to confirm if the patient prefers the axis returning to where it is expected to lie.

Oguchi's disease
A rare cause of **congenital stationary nightblindness type II**. The **fundus** appears grey. Rod **adaptation** is delayed for many hours.

OH
Acronym of ocular history.

OHT
Acronym of ***ocular hypertension.***

OK
Acronym of ***orthokeratology.***

OKAN
Acronym of ***optokinetic after-nystagmus.***

OKN
Acronym of ***optokinetic nystagmus.***

OKNd
Abbreviation of ***delayed optokinetic nystagmus.***

OKNe
Abbreviation of ***early optokinetic nystagmus.***

OKR
Acronym of ***optokinetic response.***

olivary pretectal nucleus
Located in the midbrain. Signals to each **Edinger–Westphal nucleus**. Involved in parasympathetic **pupil** size control. *Synonym is* ***pretectal nucleus.***

OLM
Acronym of ***outer limiting membrane.***

OM
Acronym of ***ocular motility.***

OMB
Acronym of ocular motor balance.

ON
Acronym of optical centre for near.

oncogene
A modified gene that increases the malignancy of a tumour cell.

oncology
The study of cancer.

one position keratometer
A **keratometer** which does not require rotating to measure both **corneal** axes. Cannot measure irregular corneal **astigmatism**. *Synonym is **variable doubling keratometer**.*

one-and-a-half syndrome
Inability to **adduct** either eye, and inability to **abduct** one eye. Indicates a lesion to the **paramedian pontine reticular formation** and **medial longitudinal fasciculus** on the side **contralateral** to the eye still able to abduct.

ONH
*Acronym of **optic nerve head**.*

OO
*Acronym of **ophthalmic optician**.*

OPAL
Acronym of occupational progressive addition lens.

open angle glaucoma
Any type of **glaucoma** in which the **anterior chamber angle** is not reduced. *Acronym is **OAG**.*

open globe
An eye with a full-thickness wound.

O

ophthalmia neonaturum
Conjunctivitis when it occurs within one month of birth.

ophthalmic nerve
The first division of the **trigeminal nerve**. Sensory nerve.

ophthalmic optician
*Synonym of **optometrist**.*

ophthalmologist
A medical specialist concerned with the diagnosis and treatment of eye disease.

ophthalmoscope
A device used to perform **ophthalmoscopy**. Note that fundus cameras and slit-lamp-based systems are not considered ophthalmoscopes, despite being used for ophthalmoscopy. *Synonym is **funduscope**.*

ophthalmoscopy
The technique of viewing the **fundus** in real-time through the **pupil**. *Synonym is **funduscopy**.*

ophthalmotrope
Mechanical device used to simulate and demonstrate anatomical insertions of the **extraocular muscles** and their actions.

OPL
*Acronym of **outer plexiform layer**.*

OPN
*Acronym of **olivary pretectal nucleus**/omnipause neuron.*

opponent theory
Theory that a colour stimulus causes an **afterimage** of its complementary colour. *Synonym is **Hering theory**.*

OPs
*Abbreviation of **oscillatory potentials**.*

opsoclonus
Ocular flutter not restricted to the horizontal plane. *Synonym is **saccadomania**.*

optic aphasia
*Synonym of **visual anomia**.*

optic array
The pattern of light reaching a point in space from all directions.

optic ataxia
Poor hand-eye coordination causing mis-reaching. Can be due to damage to parietal cortex.

optic chiasm
The point at which the optic nerves cross and **decussation** occurs; leads to the **optic tracts**. Anatomically lies above the pituitary gland. *Synonym is **chiasm**.*

optic disc
*Synonym of **optic nerve head**.*

optic disc drusen
*Synonym of **disc drusen**.*

optic disc haemorrhage
*Synonym of **splinter haemorrhage**.*

optic disc hypoplasia
*Synonym of **optic nerve hypoplasia**.*

O

optic disc pit
Coloboma in the neural retina that occurs at the temporal **disc**. No problem, unless there is a **macular** detachment. *Synonym is **optic pit**.*

optic flow
The flow of the **optic array** around the visual system.

optic foramen
Foramen through which the optic nerve passes.

optic nerve
Known as cranial nerve II, despite being myelinated and therefore not technically a cranial nerve.

optic nerve glioma
Tumour of optic nerve glial tissue. Associated with **neurofibromatosis type 1**. Causes **proptosis**. Often occurs in the young, especially in girls. Causes vision loss.

optic nerve head
Point where the optic nerve joins the eye (blind spot). Pale due to myelin sheaths. *Acronym is ONH. Synonyms are **disc**, **optic disc**, and **optic papilla**.*

optic nerve hypoplasia
Small, pink **optic disc**. Often **infantile nystagmus** and reduced visual acuity. *Synonym is **optic disc hypoplasia**.*

optic neuritis
Inflammation of the **optic nerve head**. May be a sign of multiple sclerosis. There are three classifications: **retrobulbar optic neuritis**, **papillitis**, and **neuroretinitis**.

optic papilla
*Synonym of **optic nerve head**.*

optic pit
*Synonym of **optic disc pit**.*

optic radiation
Carries information from the **lateral geniculate nucleus** to the **visual cortex** along calcarine fissure of the parietal lobe.

optic tectum
*Synonym of **superior colliculus**.*

optic tract
The optic nerve between the **optic chiasm** and **lateral geniculate nucleus**.

optical aniseikonia
Physical difference in retinal image sizes. **Neural aniseikonia** can develop to correct this.

optical centre
The point in a lens through which light passes unrefracted and undeviated. *Acronym is **OC**.*

optical character recognition
Computerised recognition of text, as used in **text-to-speech** devices as an **assistive technology**. *Acronym is **OCR**.*

optical coherence tomography
Method of assessing the individual layers of the **fundus**; uses pulses of light in similar manner to ultrasound. A few sub-types include: **swept source optical coherence tomography**, **spectral domain optical coherence tomography**, **time domain optical coherence tomography**, and **frequency domain optical coherence tomography**. *Acronym is **OCT**.*

opticociliary shunt
Dilated **collaterals** at the **optic nerve head**. May indicate optic nerve sheath **meningioma** or optic nerve **glioma**. May develop following **retinal vein occlusion**. *Synonym is **optociliary shunt**.*

optociliary shunt
*Synonym of **opticociliary shunt**.*

optogram
The image obtained by the process of **optography**.

O

optography
Chemical recovery of the image last viewed by a retina before death. The process was once purported to be useful in forensic science but since has been found to be inadequate except under controlled laboratory conditions, and virtually impossible in humans due to the tiny size of the **fovea**.

optokinetic after-nystagmus
The sustained, decelerating **nystagmus** resulting when lights are extinguished during **optokinetic nystagmus**. *Acronym is **OKAN**. Synonym is **after-nystagmus**.*

optokinetic nystagmus
Reflex eye movement in response to **retinal slip**. There are two kinds: **look optokinetic nystagmus** and **stare optokinetic nystagmus**. *Acronym is **OKN**. Synonym is **optokinetic response**.*

optokinetic response
*Synonym of **optokinetic nystagmus**.*

optometer
Any device that measures the refractive power of the eye.

optometrist
An eye care professional concerned with all aspects of spectacle and contact lens correction, **orthoptics**, and primary care for ocular health matters. *Synonym is* ***ophthalmic optician***.

optotype
Any symbol or character used in a vision testing chart, e.g. **Sloan letter**s, **Tumbling** Es, or **Landolt** Cs.

ora
Synonym of ***ora serrata***.

ora serrata
Serrated join between retina and **ciliary body**. **Retinal detachment** does not occur here. *Synonym is* ***ora***.

orbicularis oculi
Sphincter-like muscle capable of closing the eye.

orbit
One of the cavities in the skull formed by the **maxilla**, **frontal bone**, **ethmoid bone**, **sphenoid bone**, **lacrimal bone**, **zygomatic bone**, and **palatine bone**, in which each eye is located.

orbital cellulitis
Cellulitis of the non-ocular **orbit**al contents posterior to the **orbital septum**. Causes **proptosis**, pain, and **periorbital** redness. May be life threatening due to risk of intracranial spread.

O

orbital myositis
Inflammation of **periorbital** region or **extraocular muscle**s; painful. Causes **proptosis** and oedema.

orbital orbicularis
The most lateral portion of the **orbicularis oculi**.

orbital septum
Sheet of connective tissue attaching bone of the **orbit** to the **eyelid**.

orbital varices
Orbital veins may bleed or thrombose. May cause intermittent **proptosis** of the eye.

organic amblyopia
Synonym of ***toxic amblyopia***.

orientation pinwheels
Areas sensitive to varying orientations found around **blob**s of **hypercolumn**s.

ornithine
In **gyrate atrophy**, ornithine is poorly metabolised, so is found in high concentration in the blood.

orthogonal lens
A **point focal lens** which is manufactured as toric, and the prescription house only have to work spherical prescription onto the lens.

orthokeratology
The use of reverse-geometry **rigid gas permeable** contact lenses worn at night to gently reshape the **cornea**, providing a temporary solution for low to moderate levels of **myopia** that requires no contact lenses or spectacles to be worn during the day. *Acronym is **OK**. Synonym is **corneal refractive therapy**.*

orthophoria
Having no latent deviation in the alignment of the eyes (**heterophoria**).

orthoptics
The discipline in eye care dealing with binocular vision abnormalities, disorders of **motility**, and **amblyopia**.

orthoptist
An eye care professional specialised in **orthoptics**.

orthoscopic lens
A lens which is corrected for peripheral **aberrations**.

orthotropia
Having no manifest deviation in the alignment of the eyes (**strabismus**).

OS
*Acronym of **oculus sinister**.*

oscillatory potentials
Up to seven disturbances seen on the rising peak of the **b-wave** of **electroretinography**, due to the activity of **amacrine cell**s and **ganglion cell**s. *Abbreviation is **OPs**.*

oscillopsia
Perceptual disturbance in which the **visual field** appears to oscillate in a drifting fashion.

osseous ampulla
*Synonym of **ampulla**.*

Ostwalt form
A form of **point focal lens** with lowest back surface power. Not really used very often.

Ota's naevus
*Synonym of **oculodermal melanosis**.*

OTC
Acronym of over-the-counter medicine.

OU
*Acronym of **oculus utro**.*

outer limiting membrane
Müller cells join to photoreceptor inner segments by zonula adherens here. *Acronym is OLM. Synonym is **external limiting membrane**.*

outer nuclear layer
Contains the photoreceptor nuclei. Cone nuclei sit next to the **outer limiting membrane**.

outer plexiform layer
Bipolar cells and **horizontal cell**s synapse with photoreceptors here. *Acronym is **OPL**.*

overaccommodation
*Synonym of **accommodative lead**.*

overt attention
Visual attention on the **fovea**ted object (as opposed to **covert attention**).

O

oxybuprocaine
An **ester-linked anaesthetic**, routinely used by **optometrist**s. Typically available at 0.4% concentration. *Synonym is **benoxinate**.*

P

P
Abbreviation of pharmacy medicine.

P-cells
Abbreviation of ***parvo cells.***

p.r.n.
Acronym of pro re nata (as required).

pachymetry
Measurement of **central corneal thickness**.

Paget's disease
Grossly deformed skull, spine, and pelvis. Causes **myopia**. Can cause **angioid streaks**.

PAL
Acronym of progressive addition lens.

palatine bone
Found between the **maxilla** and **sphenoid bones**. Part of the roof of the mouth and floor of the **orbit**.

pale stripe
Synonym of ***interstripe.***

pallor
Paleness.

pallor-cup discrepancy
Optic nerve cupping that is more advanced than the **pallor** – suggests **glaucoma** over other pathology.

palpebra
Synonym of ***eyelid.***

palpebral
Of or relating to the **eyelids**.

palpebral aperture
Synonym of ***palpebral fissure.***

palpebral conjunctiva
Synonym of ***tarsal conjunctiva.***

palpebral fissure
The gap between the upper and lower **eyelids**. *Synonym is **palpebral aperture**.*

palpebral furrow
Crease in the **palpebral** skin, roughly at the margin of the **tarsal plate**s.

palpebral oculogyric reflex
*Synonym of **Bell's phenomenon**.*

palpitations
Unusual awareness of heart beating.

palsy
Paralysis or **paresis** of a body part accompanied by loss of feeling and uncontrolled movement.

PAM
Acronym of primary acquired melanoma.

PAN
*Acronym of **periodic alternating nystagmus**/polyarteritis nodosa.*

Pancoast tumour
Tumour of lung apex. Signs are **Horner's syndrome**, **haemoptysis**, cachexia, cough, hoarse voice, recurrent chest infections.

pannus
Abnormal vessel growth in the **cornea**.

panophthalmitis
Inflammation of the entire eye, including the **orbit**.

panretinal photocoagulation
The burning of blood vessels throughout the retina with an argon laser, e.g. in **diabetic retinopathy**. *Acronym is **PRP**.*

pantoscopic tilt
The extent to which the top of a pair of spectacles is tilted away from the patient's face.

Panum's fusional area
The area around the **horopter** over which, if an image is seen by both eyes, **fusion** will occur. Outside this area **diplopia** occurs. The area is larger in the periphery.

panuveitis
Inflammation of the entire **uvea**.

papilla
*Singular of **papillae**.*

papillae
Nodular swellings of the **tarsal conjunctiva** with a central vascular tuft due to **inflammation**. *Singular is **papilla**.*

papillary conjunctivitis
*Synonym of **contact lens induced papillary conjunctivitis**.*

papillitis
Optic neuritis restricted to the **optic nerve head** – causes enlarged blind spot and central **visual field** defect.

papilloedema
Non-inflammatory swelling of the **optic nerve head** due to increased intracranial pressure (possibly cerebral tumour); usually bilateral. Causes **macular star** and **Paton's lines**. May cause headache.

papilloma
Skin growth, often found on the **eyelid** or **conjunctiva**. Usually benign; can be removed with cryotherapy.

paradoxical anomalous retinal correspondence
Anomalous retinal correspondence in which the patient is aware of a **strabismus**, and the magnitude is greater than the objective angle of deviation.

parafovea
Area around the **fovea**, within the **perifovea**.

parahippocampal place area
Brain region medial to the **fusiform face area**. Encodes visual information about places and landmarks.

parallax
The perceived displacement of the orientation and position of an object when it is viewed from different angles. When viewing an object **monocular**ly (e.g. in direct **ophthalmoscopy**), this provides depth cues.

paramedian pontine reticular formation
The horizontal **saccade** control centre. Located in the pons. *Acronym is **PPRF**.*

pareidolia
Phenomenon in which a non-meaningful stimulus elicits a mistaken perception; e.g. perception of a face in a cloud.

paresis
Underaction of a muscle; a partial paralysis. *Synonym is **paretic**.*

paretic
*Synonym of **paresis**.*

P

parietal stream
Synonym of ***dorsal stream.***

Parinaud–Koerber–Salus–Elschnig syndrome
Synonym of ***dorsal midbrain syndrome.***

Parinaud's syndrome
Synonym of ***dorsal midbrain syndrome.***

Parks three-step test
Algorithmic method to determine which **extraocular muscle** is **paretic**: (1) find the eye with **hypertropia** (either the **depressors** in that eye, or **elevators** of the other are responsible); (2) determine if **diplopia** is worse in **dextroversion** or **laevoversion** (indicates either the vertical recti of the eye on that side, or obliques of the other); and (3) perform the **Bielschowsky head tilt test**. *Synonym is* ***Parks–Bielschowsky three-step test.***

Parks–Bielschowsky three-step test
Synonym of ***Parks three-step test.***

pars plicata
Anterior section of the **ciliary body**, in front of the **ora serrata**. Ridged (plicated).

parvo cells
Cells that represent a part of the **parvocellular pathway**. *Abbreviation is* ***P-cells.*** *Synonyms are* ***midget cells*** *and* ***tonic cells.***

parvocellular pathway
The sub-pathway of the visual system containing information about colour, high **contrast**, and high resolution stimuli.

P

PAS
Acronym of palpebral aperture size/peripheral ***anterior synechiae.***

Paton's lines
Radial lines about the temporal **optic nerve head** in **papilloedema**.

pattern deviation map
On a **perimetry** printout, the rightmost difference diagram. Allows for analysis of the shape of the **visual field**.

pattern electroretinogram
Primarily assesses **macular** function. Contains two components: the pattern-specific response and retinal **illuminance** response. *Acronym is* ***PERG.***

pattern glare
Synonym of ***visual stress.***

pattern onset/offset electroretinogram
Electroretinography using a checkerboard pattern in which both the light and dark squares fade to grey and back again. This overall equal luminance means that scattered light does not become a confounding factor in the analysis.

pattern reversal electroretinogram
Electroretinography using an alternating-luminance checkerboard pattern: achieves electroretinography without scattered light being a problem.

pattern standard deviation
In **perimetry**, the standard deviation of the difference of each deviation from the expected value for that patient. Measured in decibels. *Acronym is* ***PSD****.*

pavingstone degeneration
Synonym of ***progressive chorioretinal atrophy****.*

PC
Acronym of post cibum (after meals).

PCA
Acronym of ***posterior cortical atrophy****.*

PCO
Acronym of ***posterior capsular opacification****.*

PCT
Acronym of prism cover test.

PD
Acronym of ***interpupillary distance****.*

PDR
Acronym of ***proliferative diabetic retinopathy****.*

PDS
Acronym of ***pigment dispersion syndrome****.*

PDT
Acronym of ***photodynamic therapy****.*

Pearson and Robinson valley detector
Mathematical model for detecting lines in a visual scene. Useful for faces, where edges aren't so useful.

PED
Acronym of ***pigment epithelium detachment****.*

P

pedicle
The synaptic terminal of cone cells. Possess many synaptic clefts. Each pedicle synapses with two **horizontal cell**s and at least two **bipolar cell**s.

peduncular hallucinosis
Complex hallucinations occurring in **scotopic** conditions. Patients often have an inverted sleep/wake cycle and/or dementia. *Synonym is **Lhermitte's hallucinosis**.*

pedunculated
Supported by a stalk.

PEE
Acronym of punctate epithelial erosion.

Peli lens
An **expansion prism** system consisting of large prisms placed above and/or below the **optical centre** of a spectacle lens, such that patients can view parts of their lost **visual field** by looking through the prism(s). The prism base is in the direction of the **hemianopia**.

Pelizaeus–Merzbacher disease
Rare inherited neurological condition causing **nystagmus**.

Pellucid degeneration
*Synonym of **Pellucid marginal degeneration**.*

Pellucid marginal degeneration
Inferior peripheral **corneal ectasia**, causing **astigmatism**. Occurs in 20–40-year-olds. Rare. *Synonym is **Pellucid degeneration**.*

pelopsia
Perceptual distortion causing objects to appear closer than they are. *Opposite is **teleopsia**.*

pencil
A group of rays.

penetrance
The extent to which a characteristic is controlled by genes in **contrast** to the environment.

penetrating keratoplasty
Keratoplasty in which the entire **cornea** is replaced. *Acronym is **PK**.*

Pentacam
A type of modern **cornea**l topographer – uses a **Scheimpflug camera**. Also used for **pachymetry**.

perceptual span
In reading research, the number/spatial extent of letters that, at any one time, contribute to reading speed. Compare with **visual attention span** and **visual span**.

Percival lens
A type of **best form lens** – free from mean oblique error but suffers from **oblique astigmatism**.

Percival's criterion
Prism required = ⅓(greater **blur point**) – ⅔(lesser blur point). Used to calculate required prism in either **eso** or **exo** deviations (only if the result of the equation is positive).

PERG
Acronym of ***pattern electroretinogram***.

peri-ballast
Synonym of ***peripheral ballast***.

peri-primary range
The ~40° of the **oculomotor range** over which the majority of eye movements occur.

peribulbar
Around the **globe**(s).

pericyte
A cell that can differentiate into a **fibroblast,** macrophage, or smooth muscle cell.

perifovea
Area around the **parafovea**, within the **macula**.

perimeter
Synonym of ***perimetry***.

perimetry
Any method for assessing the **visual field**. This may involve **static perimetry** or **kinetic perimetry** principles, and can be practitioner-controlled or automated. *Synonym is* ***perimeter***.

perinatal
Time around birth.

periodic alternating nystagmus
Nystagmus with a **nystagmus waveform** that varies with time. Cycles are typically between one and four minutes; in this time there may be periods of jerk right, jerk left, and pendular nystagmus.

periorbital
Around the **orbit**.

peripapillary atrophy
Stretching of the **posterior pole**, resulting in drag of the **choroid** and **retinal pigment epithelium**, leaving a **temporal crescent** from the **optic nerve head**. *Acronym is PPA*.

P

peripapillary staphyloma
Cause a normal looking **optic disc** but with peripapillary excavation.

peripheral ballast
Similar to the prism ballast design of contact lens stabilisation, except that the prism only exists in the lens periphery – not the optic zone. *Synonym is **peri-ballast**.*

peripheral drusen
Hard drusen or **soft drusen** found near the equator of the eye due to build-up of **retinal pigment epithelium** waste products. Does not necessarily indicate **macular degeneration**, although those with **AMD** are more likely to have peripheral drusen.

peripheral iridotomy
Holes punctured in the peripheral iris by laser, usually to increase aqueous drainage in **glaucoma** patients. *Acronym is **PI**.*

peripheral nystagmus
Any **nystagmus** originating from the vestibular system (i.e. nystagmus that cannot be described as **central nystagmus**).

peripheral ulcerative keratitis
May be caused by collagen disorders; polyarteritis nodosa, rheumatoid arthritis, Wegener's granulomatosis. *Acronym is **PUK**.*

periphlebitis
Inflammation of a vein wall.

periscopic lens
A meniscus lens with a ±1.25 D surface.

Perkins tonometer
A handheld portable **applanation tonometer**, useful in a domiciliary setting or for uncooperative patients and those who cannot physically sit at a slit lamp. Probe diameter is 3.06 mm. Similar in principle to the **Goldmann tonometer**.

PERLA
Acronym of pupils equal, reacting to light and accommodation.

PERRL
Acronym of pupils equal, round, and reacting to light.

persistent foetal vessels
*Synonym of **persistent hyperplastic primary vitreous**.*

persistent hyperplastic primary vitreous
A mass remnant of the **primary vitreous** from embryonic development. Causes **leukocoria** and **lens opacity**. *Acronym is **PHPV**. Synonym is **persistent foetal vessels**.*

PET
Acronym of positron emission tomography.

Peter's anomaly
Congenital **corneal** opacification and either **anterior synechia** or keratolenticular adhesion. Associated with **buphthalmos.**

Petit's canal
The space between the posterior **zonules of Zinn** and the **vitreous humour**. *Synonym is **canal of Petit**.*

Petzval lens
*Synonym of **point focal lens**.*

Petzval surface
The 'curvature of field' **aberration**. Has no astigmatic error. **Point focal lens**es focus on this.

PFV
*Acronym of **persistent foetal vessels/positive fusional vergence**.*

phacodonesis
Vibration of the crystalline lens during eye movements, usually due to **lens subluxation**.

phacoemulsification
The process of emulsifying the lens with an ultrasound probe in **cataract** extraction.

phacolytic glaucoma
Secondary **glaucoma** due to debris from **phacolytic uveitis** blocking the **trabecular meshwork**.

phacolytic uveitis
Uveitis secondary to a **Morgagnian cataract**.

phacomorphic glaucoma
Glaucoma caused by **pupillary block** due to an **intumescent cataract.**

phakic intraocular lens
An **intraocular lens** that is used whilst the natural crystalline lens is still in place. *Acronym is **pIOL**.*

phantom array effect
Illusory perception of multiple discrete lights seen when making a **saccade** across a temporally modulated light source.

phantom eye syndrome
Hallucinatory **globe** pain and **Charles Bonnet syndrome** following **enucleation.**

phantopsia
Visual **hallucination**.

pharmacodynamics
The study of the effect of drugs on the body, the methods of action, and effects of dose.

pharmacogenomics
The concept of designing drugs to the patient's specific genetic make-up.

pharyngoconjunctival fever
An upper respiratory tract infection caused by **adenovirus**, usually in children. **Keratitis** in 30% of cases.

pharyngotympanic tube
Links the ear to the **pharynx**. Equalises pressure and drains mucus.

pharynx
The tube that connects the mouth, nose, and oesophagus.

phasic cells
*Synonym of **magno cells**.*

phasing
The practice of taking multiple **tonometry** readings throughout a day to monitor changes in **intraocular pressure**; usually requires hospital admission.

PHE
*Acronym of **phenylephrine**.*

phenol red test
Cotton with a pH indicator is placed a third of the distance from the temporal **canthus** in the lower **fornix**. The length of cotton that turns yellow within 15 seconds is measured. <9 mm indicates dry eye syndrome. *Synonym is **cotton thread test**.*

phenylephrine
A sympathomimetic **mydriatic**. Typically available in 5% and 10% concentrations. *Acronym is **PHE**.*

phi motion
Apparent motion caused by successive removal of adjacent stimuli. Causes the appearance of a stimulus in the moving gap that has no shape.

phi test
A modified cover test in which the patient is asked to give a subjective report of perceived image movement.

phlycten
Inflammatory nodule on the **bulbar conjunctiva**, surrounded by **hyperaemia**. Due to delayed hypersensitivity to an antigen (usually staphylococcus). *Synonyms are* ***phlyctenular keratoconjunctivitis*** *and* ***phlyctenulosis***.

phlyctenular keratoconjunctivitis
Synonym of ***phlycten***.

phlyctenulosis
Synonym of ***phlycten***.

PhNR
Abbreviation of ***photopic negative response***.

phoria
Synonym of ***heterophoria***.

phoria method
Method of calculating **accommodative convergence:accommodation ratio.** Formula: **interpupillary distance** + (near **heterophoria** – distance heterophoria)/**accommodation** demand of near target. **Eso** deviations are positive; **exo** are negative. *Synonym is* ***heterophoria method***.

phoropter
Device containing an array of lenses which can be positioned in various combinations in front of each eye to perform a **refraction**.

phosphene
The perception of light when no light source exists.

photodynamic therapy
Treatment for **choroidal neovascularisation.** Following **intravitreal** injection of **verteporfin** and a wait of 15 minutes, a light is shone into the eye which causes activation of the verteporfin which collects in rapidly dividing cells (the site of **neovascularisation**). *Acronym is PDT. Synonym is* ***verteporfin photodynamic therapy***.

photogenous asthenopia
Asthenopia caused by glare.

photokeratitis
Painful **keratitis** caused by intense UV-B light, e.g. arc welding. *Synonyms are* ***arc-eye*** *and* ***snow blindness***.

photon
Quantum of light energy.

photophobia
Abnormal aversion to light.

P

photopic
High **illumination** levels in which cones are responsive but rods are not.

photopic negative response
In **electroretinography**, a negative wave due to **ganglion cell** activity. *Abbreviation is **PhNR**.*

photopsia
Perception of flashing lights/sparks/colours. Suggests **posterior vitreous detachment** or **retinal detachment**. *Plural is **photopsiae**.*

photopsiae
*Plural of **photopsia**.*

photorefractive keratectomy
The **corneal epithelium** is removed with alcohol/blade. Stroma is ablated, and the epithelium eventually grows back. *Acronym is **PRK**. Synonym is **advanced surface ablation**.*

photoscopy
*Synonym of **retinoscopy**.*

photostress test
Bleach **macula** for 30 seconds with light; the time taken before patient can see one line less than their best **visual acuity** again is measured. Greater than one minute is considered pathological. *Synonym is **light stress test**.*

PHPV
*Acronym of **persistent hyperplastic primary vitreous**.*

phthisis bulbi
Microphthalmos due to shrinkage/atrophy of the **globe** following severe disease/ **inflammation**.

physiological anisocoria
Anisocoria <1 mm. Present in ~20% of the population.

physiological diplopia
Diplopia experienced when an object lies outside of **Panum's fusional area**. Completely normal.

physiological suppression
Suppression of one of the physiological **diplopia** images, usually of the non-dominant eye.

physiological V-pattern
The fact that some **convergence** is normal in **depression**.

PI
*Acronym of **peripheral iridotomy**.*

pia mater
The innermost **meninx**, very thin and delicate.

PIC
Acronym of pseudoisochromatic plates.

Pickford–Nicolson anomaloscope
A type of **anomaloscope** that is no longer in use.

pigment dispersion syndrome
Occurs when the **zonules of Zinn** rub the posterior iris, causing pigment to float in the **anterior chamber**, which can block the **trabecular meshwork**, leading to **pigmentary glaucoma**. Can cause a **Krukenberg spindle** to form. *Acronym is **PDS**.*

pigment epithelium detachment
Detachment of the **retinal pigment epithelium**. *Acronym is **PED**.*

pigmentary glaucoma
Glaucoma following **pigment dispersion syndrome**, due to **aqueous humour** outflow being impeded by the blocked **trabecular meshwork**. This causes a rise in **intraocular pressure**.

pilocarpine
A parasympathomimetic **miotic**. Typically available at 0.5% concentration.

pinguecula
Calcification and collagen in the sub-epithelial **bulbar conjunctiva**. Appearance is as a raised yellow-white oval. A normal finding found in most individuals to some degree; extent depends largely on ultraviolet light exposure. Occurs to a greater extent on the nasal side as light hits the temporal **cornea** and is totally internally reflected to end up at the nasal **conjunctiva**.

pIOL
*Acronym of **phakic intraocular lens**.*

Piper's law of spatial summation
For an area larger than a **receptive field**, luminance threshold multiplied by the square root of the stimulus size is constant.

pitch
Describes a head turn in the up-down axis (nodding of the head in this axis would usually be interpreted as 'yes').

PK
*Acronym of **penetrating keratoplasty**.*

PL
*Acronym of perception of light/**preferential looking test**.*

Placido disc
A series of concentric rings used in **corneal** topographers to provide a reflection reference.

Planckian locus
The path taken by a **black body** at varying temperatures on the CIE diagram. *Synonym is* ***black body curve***.

plaque
Drusen (usually larger).

plastic period
The time in which there is **cortical** plasticity. Varies for different areas of the brain. *Synonym is* ***critical period***.

pleomorphic adenoma
Onset in the 4th–5th decades of life. Painless slow-growing tumour in the **lacrimal fossa**. **Globe** displaced.

pleomorphism
Synonym of ***polymorphism***.

pleoptics
The technique of dazzling an **eccentric fixation** point whilst protecting the **fovea** from light, in the hope that the fovea will take up **fixation**.

plica semilunaris
Vestigial fold of the **conjunctiva** found next to the **lacrimal caruncle**, formerly the nictating membrane.

P

PLTF
Acronym of pre-lens tear film.

plus disease
A variant of **retinopathy of prematurity** – a sign of **ischaemia**. Rigid **pupil**, vitreal haze, peripheral **telangiectasia**.

plus lens
A convex lens that causes light to become more convergent/less divergent.

PMD
*Acronym of Pelizaeus–Merzbacher disease/****Pellucid marginal degeneration***.

PMMA
Acronym of ***poly(methyl methacrylate)***.

PMR
Acronym of ***polymyalgia rheumatica***.

pneumatic retinopexy
External compression applied to reattach the retina surgically.

pneumatic vitreolysis
Intravitreal injection of gas, used as a treatment to release focal **vitreomacular traction**.

pneumocystis carinii pneumonia
Condition that only tends to occur in immuno-compromised patients; a common sign of AIDS.

PNS
Acronym of peripheral nervous system.

PO
Acronym of per os (orally).

POAG
Acronym of ***primary open angle glaucoma****.*

POBF
Acronym of ***pulsatile ocular blood flow****.*

POH
Acronym of previous ocular history.

point focal lens
A type of **best form lens** – free from **oblique astigmatism** but suffers from mean oblique error. *Synonym is* ***Petzval lens****.*

point spread function
The amount that an optical system blurs a point source.

point zero
In **strabismus**, the part of the retina looking at the same object as the **fovea** of the other.

polariser
Removes electric fields in all directions except one.

polarographic method
International standard for measuring Dk of soft lenses of Dk <100. *Synonym is* ***Fatt method****.*

poliosis
Greying/whitening of hair.

poly(methyl methacrylate)
Material from which hard contact lenses were once made. *Acronym is* ***PMMA****.*

P

polycoria
Multiple **pupil**s (openings of the iris) in one eye – iridotomies only count if particularly large.

polymegethism
Corneal endothelium cells are different sizes. Due to **hypoxia**.

polymorphism
The case in which **corneal endothelium** cells are different shapes. Due to **hypoxia**. *Synonym is pleomorphism.*

polymyalgia rheumatica
Pain and stiffness in neck, shoulders, and hips, worse in the morning. Associated with **giant cell arteritis**. *Acronym is PMR.*

polymyxin B
An antibacterial. Effective against **pseudomonas**.

polynomial aspheric
A lens used to correct high **ametropia**, with a similar approach to a **lenticular lens**, but in which the power is changed gradually towards the periphery to reduce thickness and weight. Field of view is therefore still sacrificed, but not as dramatically as in a lenticular lens.

polyopia
The perception of multiple images (like **diplopia**, but more images).

polyquad
A high molecular weight preservative found in some contact lens solutions.

P

polytrichosis
Excessive hair growth. In the eyes, refers to an excessive number of **lash**es.

PoM
Acronym of prescription-only medicine.

Ponzo illusion
Visual illusion which uses perspective perception to cause two lines of the same length to appear different (a capital 'A' shape with two horizontal beams; the lower of the two appears shorter).

porropsia
A form of **hallucination** in which objects appear to be moving away from the observer without changing in size.

positional nystagmus
A type of **vestibular nystagmus** induced by placing the head in a specific position. Can be caused by **benign paroxysmal positional vertigo**.

positive fusional reserve
The **fusional reserve** measured using base out prism. *Synonym is **convergence fusional reserve**.*

positive fusional vergence
The **fusional vergence** limit in response to base out prism.

positive relative accommodation
The amount of negative spherical power that can be added to the initial reading **addition** before blur/**diplopia** is perceived. *Acronym is **PRA**.*

positive retinal disparity
*Synonym of **crossed retinal disparity**.*

positive vertical vergence
Right eye rotates higher than left.

Posner–Schlossman syndrome
Recurrent **anterior uveitis** which can lead to a secondary **glaucoma**. *Synonym is **glaucomatocyclitic crisis**.*

post-operative consecutive esotropia
A **consecutive esotropia** occurring following surgery to an **extraocular muscle**.

post-operative consecutive exotropia
A **consecutive exotropia** occurring following surgery to an **extraocular muscle**.

post-operative diplopia test
Prism used to find out how much disparity causes **diplopia**, to estimate the effect of over/undercorrection in surgery on binocularity.

post-saccadic oscillation
Distortion of the **pupil** margin and displacement of the crystalline lens that occurs following a **saccade**. Caused by the elasticity of the ocular contents and laxity of the **zonules of Zinn**. Noticeable in the output of high speed video-based **eye trackers**.

posterior blepharitis
Blepharitis: specifically, **inflammation** of the **meibomian glands**.

posterior capsular opacification
Either **Elschnig pearl** or **capsular phimosis** that occurs following **cataract** surgery, causing the **lens capsule** to become opaque. Treated by **capsulotomy**. *Acronym is **PCO**.*

posterior chamber
Small chamber between the iris and **zonules of Zinn**.

P

posterior cortical atrophy
Unusual presentation of Alzheimer's disease causing **visual agnosia**s. *Acronym is* ***PCA***. *Synonym is* ***Benson's syndrome***.

posterior embryotoxon
Congenital defect, an opaque line showing thickening of **Schwalbe's line**.

posterior lenticonus
Abnormal bulge in the posterior lens that can develop in early childhood.

posterior pole
The point where the geometric **axis** of the eye crosses the posterior surface(s).

posterior polymorphous dystrophy
Posterior **cornea**l dystrophy. Asymptomatic. Subtle geographical/band-like **lesion**s. *Acronym is* ***PPD***.

posterior staphyloma
Bulge at the back of the eye in pathological **myopia**.

posterior subcapsular cataract
Cataract that causes poorer vision than a more anterior cataract (as it is situated closer to the nodal point of the eye). Often caused by steroid use, diabetes, and **gyrate atrophy**. More common in men. *Synonym is* ***posterior subcapsular lens opacity***.

posterior subcapsular lens opacity
Synonym of ***posterior subcapsular cataract***.

P

posterior synechia
Adhesion of the iris to the lens. *Acronym is* ***PS***.

posterior uvea
The **uveal** tract behind the posterior border of the **vitreous** base.

posterior uveitis
Inflammation of the **posterior uvea**.

posterior vitreous detachment
Condition in which the **vitreous humour** detaches from the retina at the back of the eye. Often causes a **Weiss ring** to appear and can cause symptoms of **photopsiae** and **floaters**. *Acronym is* ***PVD***. *General form is* ***vitreous detachment***.

postfixed chiasm
The situation in which the **optic chiasm** is posterior to the pituitary gland.

postganglionic nerve cell
An autonomic nerve fibre from ganglion to effector organ.

POTF
Acronym of pre-ocular tear film.

Pourfour du Petit syndrome
Pupil abnormality causing the inverse effects of **Horner's syndrome** due to excitation of nerves by encroaching tumour. Further compression by tumour often leads to **Horner's pupil**.

power rings
In high powered negative lenses, the ring effect seen when looking obliquely at the lens edge.

PPA
Acronym of ***peripapillary atrophy****.*

PPD
Acronym of ***posterior polymorphous dystrophy****.*

PPDR
Acronym of ***pre-proliferative diabetic retinopathy****.*

PPE
Acronym of personal protective equipment.

PPRF
Acronym of ***paramedian pontine reticular formation****.*

PPV
Acronym of pars plana ***vitrectomy****.*

PR
Acronym of photoreceptor.

PRA
Acronym of ***positive relative accommodation****.*

pre-auricular depression
Dip in the skull **ventral** to the ear – used as a reference point when attaching electrodes.

pre-eclampsia
Hypertension and proteinuria in late pregnancy – can cause a **serous retinal detachment**.

pre-proliferative diabetic retinopathy
Intraretinal microvascular abnormalities, cotton wool spots, dark **blot haemorrhages**, venous irregularities. *Acronym is* ***PPDR****.*

P

precision vision 16
Colour vision test similar to the **Farnsworth D15 test**, but chunkier pieces which are laminated. For children. *Abbreviation is **PV-16**.*

preferential looking test
Any test of the visual system designed for use with uncomprehending patients in which two stimuli are presented simultaneously causing the patient to be (in theory) compelled to view the more visually stimulating of the two. The practitioner must decide in which direction the patient initially looked to assess whether they can truly resolve the stimulus or not.

preferred retinal locus
The area of retina used for **eccentric viewing** when a patient has a central **scotoma**. *Acronym is **PRL**.*

prefixed chiasm
The situation in which the **optic chiasm** is anterior to the pituitary gland.

preganglionic nerve cell
An autonomic nerve fibre from the central nervous system to ganglion.

Prentice's rule
Formula used to calculate the amount of prismatic effect induced upon light rays travelling through a non-central point of a lens: $P = cF$; where P = prism dioptres, c = distance from optical centre (in cm), F = power of lens (in D).

preretinal haemorrhage
A haemorrhage between the **vitreous humour** and the retina. Appears as having a flat top.

preretinal membrane
*Synonym of **epiretinal membrane**.*

presbyope
An individual with **presbyopia**.

presbyopia
Gradual loss of **accommodation** due to the continued growth of the lens causing a loss of elasticity.

preseptal orbicularis
The **orbicularis oculi** between the **pretarsal orbicularis** and **orbital orbicularis**.

presumed ocular histoplasmosis syndrome
Fungal infection, asymptomatic. **Fundus** lesions, **choroidal neovascularisation**, **peripapillary atrophy**. *Synonym is **ocular histoplasmosis**.*

pretarsal orbicularis
The **orbicularis oculi** between the **preseptal orbicularis** and **marginal orbicularis**.

pretectal nucleus
Synonym of ***olivary pretectal nucleus.***

prevalence
The number of people in a population with a disease at any given time. Compare with **incidence**.

primal sketch
The pre-attentive sketch in the brain similar to that produced by the **Marr–Hildreth computational model**.

primary acquired melanosis
Hyperpigmented area of **conjunctiva** (tumour). Often patients are elderly. Atypical cells indicate malignancy.

primary decompensated microtropia
A **microtropia** that has increased in size due to **Lang's esopetal factors**.

primary deviation
In **strabismus**, the ocular deviation angle when fixating with the non-strabismic eye.

primary eye care
The first point of contact for the public to eye care services, e.g. as provided by an **optometrist**.

primary familial amyloidosis
Synonym of ***gelatinous drop-like dystrophy.***

primary headache
Any form of **headache** which does not occur secondary to some other condition.

primary hypertension
Synonym of ***essential hypertension.***

primary Jones test
Cotton bud is placed in the nose, and **sodium fluorescein** is instilled onto the eye. The transmission of dye onto the bud indicates **nasolacrimal duct** patency. *Synonym is* ***Jones I test.***

primary microtropia
Microtropia in which the microtropia was the initial defect (not caused by anything else).

primary open angle glaucoma
Open angle glaucoma not due to **pigmentary glaucoma**. *Acronym is* ***POAG.***

primary position
Describes a straight-ahead position of **gaze**.

P

primary visual cortex

Area of the brain that synapses with **optic radiation**s from the **lateral geniculate nucleus**, located in the **occipital lobe** of the brain. *Synonyms are **Brodmann area 17**, **striate cortex**, and **V1**.*

primary vitreous

The type of **vitreous humour** present during embryonic development. Formed by the rim of the optic cup. Later displaced by the **secondary vitreous**.

prion

A proteinous infectious particle, only made of protein, e.g. Creutzfeldt–Jakob disease.

PRIS

Acronym of photoreceptor inner segment.

prism ballast

Method of contact lens stabilisation. Base down prism is built into the lens, which weights down the lens, reducing spontaneous rotation.

prism dioptre

A measure of angular deviation of light; can be used to infer the size of an ocular deviation, although technically it refers to the correction required. One prism dioptre is one unit of angular deviation at a distance of 100 units; e.g. a beam of light that is deviated five centimetres when shone at a distance of one metre is deviated by five prism dioptres. $7\ \Delta \approx 4°$.

prisoner's cinema

Intrinsic light, **entoptic phenomena**, and **hallucination**s reported to occur following prolonged sensory deprivation.

P

PRK

*Acronym of **photorefractive keratectomy**.*

PRL

*Acronym of **preferred retinal locus**.*

progressive chorioretinal atrophy

Enlarged **globe** causing almost bare **sclera** at the **fundus**. May be associated with **macular hole**s. *Synonyms are **cobblestone degeneration**, **cobblestone retinopathy**, and **pavingstone degeneration**.*

progressive esotropia fixus

*Synonym of **heavy eye syndrome**.*

progressive external ophthalmoplegia

Bilateral loss of eye movement. **Ptosis**, **diplopia**.

progressive supranuclear palsy
Neurodegenerative condition causing loss of proprioception. Initial vertical gaze palsy; later horizontal. Dementia. *Acronym is **PSP**. Synonym is **Steele–Richardson–Olszewski syndrome**.*

progressor
A computer programme used to show change in **visual fields** over time by comparing the linear **regression** of each visual field position over time.

prolate
Describes a curve that flattens in the periphery.

proliferation
Division (in cells).

proliferative diabetic retinopathy
Haemorrhages, **posterior vitreous detachment**, **neovascularisation** of the **optic disc**, **new vessels elsewhere**. *Acronym is **PDR**.*

proliferative sickle cell retinopathy
Sea-fan neovascularisation, haemorrhaging, fibrovascular **proliferation**.

pronase
An enzyme tablet for contact lens cleaning.

propamidine
An antibacterial. **Pseudomonas** is resistant. *Synonym is **brolene**.*

proprioception
The sense of where parts of one's body are.

proptosis
A bulging of the eye anteriorly out of the **orbit**. Causes **Dalrymple's sign**. Measured using a **Hertel exophthalmometer**. *Synonym is **exophthalmos**.*

PROS
Acronym of photoreceptor outer segment.

prosaccade
The opposite of an **antisaccade**; i.e. a **saccade** made towards a target.

prosopagnosia
Inability to recognise faces. A specific type of **visual agnosia**. There are two types: **apperceptive prosopagnosia** and **associative prosopagnosia**.

prosopometamorphopsia
Distorted perception of faces and facial expressions.

P

prosthetic contact lens
A vague term, used to refer to contact lenses that change the appearance of the eye.

prostitute's pupil
Synonym of ***Argyll Robertson pupil.***

protan
Refers to both **protanope**s and **protanomalope**s.

protanomalope
An individual with a **protanomaly**.

protanomaly
Anomalous trichromatism in which more red is required for colour matching.

protanope
An individual with a **protanopia**.

protanopia
Dichromatism in which there is no **erythrolabe** pigment.

proximal accommodation
Accommodation caused by the knowledge that an object is close.

proximal convergence
Convergence caused by the knowledge that an object is close.

P

proxymetacaine
An **ester-linked anaesthetic**, routinely used by **optometrist**s. Typically available at 0.5% concentration, and with **fluorescein** for **applanation tonometry**. *Acronym is* ***PRX.***

PRP
Acronym of ***panretinal photocoagulation.***

pruritus
Itch.

PRX
Acronym of ***proxymetacaine.***

PS
Acronym of ***posterior synechia.***

PSCLO
Acronym of ***posterior subcapsular lens opacity.***

PSD
Acronym of ***pattern standard deviation.***

PSE
Acronym of point of subjective equality.

pseudoesotropia
The appearance of an **esotropia** when no such deviation exists; often caused by large **epicanthal folds** giving the appearance that the eyes are turned in.

pseudoexfoliation syndrome
Bits of amyloid material float in the **anterior chamber** and stick to the anterior lens and **trabecular meshwork**. Leads to **pseudoexfoliative glaucoma**. *Acronyms are PXF and PXS. Synonym is* ***exfoliation syndrome.***

pseudoexfoliative glaucoma
Glaucoma caused by **pseudoexfoliation syndrome**.

pseudohallucination
A **hallucination** that the observer recognises as not real.

pseudomonas
Synonym of ***pseudomonas aeruginosa.***

pseudomonas aeruginosa
An uncommon **Gram-negative** bacterial infection. Penetrates the **cornea** fast; can cause **retinal detachment**. Resistant to **chloramphenicol** and **propamidine**. *Synonym is* ***pseudomonas.***

pseudoneglect
Phenomenon whereby most normally sighted individuals show a small leftward bias when performing line bisection tasks; as if they have a mild form of left **unilateral neglect**.

pseudopapilloedema
The false appearance of **papilloedema**. May be caused by a small **optic nerve head**, buried **drusen**, a **crowded disc, myelinated nerve fibres**, a **tilted disc**, or tumour.

pseudophake
An individual with an **intraocular lens** implant of any type.

pseudophakic bullous keratopathy
Dystrophia epithelialis corneae with **corneal epithelium** oedema as a complication of **cataract** extraction.

pseudoproptosis
Eyelid retraction, giving appearance of **proptosis** (e.g. in **Graves' disease**).

P

pseudostrabismus
The false appearance of **strabismus** due to **epicanthal fold**s or facial asymmetry.

pseudostratified
That which appears to be **stratified** but is not.

pseudotumour cerebri
Synonym of ***idiopathic intracranial hypertension****.*

pseudoxanthoma elasticum
An inherited connective tissue disease; causes **myopia**. Can cause **angioid streaks**. *Acronym is PXE.*

PSNS
Acronym of parasympathetic nervous system.

PSP
Acronym of ***progressive supranuclear palsy****.*

PSR
Acronym of pattern-specific response.

PSRT
Acronym of photostress test recovery time.

psychiatric headache
A generalised headache with vague symptoms.

psychogenic flutter
Synonym of ***voluntary nystagmus****.*

psychological nystagmus
Synonym of ***voluntary nystagmus****.*

psychometric function
In **psychophysics**, a graph showing frequency of perception against stimulus intensity.

psychophysical
Adjective form of ***psychophysics****.*

psychophysics
Scientific discipline involving the measurement of perception. Often achieved through the **classical psychophysical methods**, **staircase method**, Bayesian or maximum likelihood estimation methods. *Adjective form is* ***psychophysical****.*

psychosensory pupillary reflex
Changes in **pupil** diameter due to emotional state. Under sympathetic and parasympathetic control, e.g. seeing an object of interest causes sympathetic **mydriasis**.

PTC
Acronym of ***pseudotumour cerebri.***

pterygia
Plural of ***pterygium.***

pterygium
A growth that can cross the **limbus**. Often bilateral. Can reappear after surgical removal. *Plural is* ***pterygia.***

PTFE
Acronym of polytetrafluoroethylene.

PTK
Acronym of phototherapeutic keratectomy.

ptosis
Abnormal drooping of the upper **eyelid**.

ptosis crutch
Synonym of ***ptosis shelf.***

ptosis prop
An attachment to spectacles that holds an **eyelid** with **ptosis** up. *Synonym is* ***Lundhi loop.***

ptosis shelf
A protrusion that can be incorporated into a scleral lens to hold the upper **eyelid** up in cases of **ptosis**. *Synonym is* ***ptosis crutch.***

PUK
Acronym of ***peripheral ulcerative keratitis.***

Pulfrich effect
False depth perception of a moving stimulus due to mismatched processing times at each retina. Can be induced by placing a neutral density filter in front of one eye, or can occur as a result of pathology such as **optic neuritis** or **cataract**.

Pulsair
A **non-contact tonometer** that uses an air puff and measures the air pressure to find **intraocular pressure**.

P

pulsatile ocular blood flow
Estimation of ocular blood flow derived from the variation in **intraocular pressure** observed during **tonometry**. *Acronym is* ***POBF.***

pulse step innervation
Describes the burst of action potentials required to initiate a **saccade**.

pulvinar
Part of the thalamus; receives input from the **superior colliculus**.

puncta
Plural of ***punctum***.

punctal stenosis
Narrowing of the **nasolacrimal duct** opening.

punctate keratitis
Keratitis which displays itself as a series of small **lesion**s.

punctum
The opening to the **canaliculus**. There are two on each eye (upper and lower **eyelid**). *Plural is* ***puncta***.

punctum proximum
Synonym of ***near point of accommodation***.

punctum remotum
The far point of the relaxed eye.

pupil
The opening in the centre of the iris.

pupil intelligence contact lens
A **multifocal contact lens** with concentric design. Zone powers reflect the normal tasks usually performed at those **pupil** sizes.

pupillary block
Condition in which the lens prevents **aqueous humour** moving to the **anterior chamber**. A pressure gradient is thus set up, causing the iris to move forward (**iris bombé**), blocking the **trabecular meshwork**, and leading to **closed angle glaucoma**.

pupillary distance
Synonym of ***interpupillary distance***.

pupillary margin
The edge of the **pupil**.

pupillary ruff
The inside edge of the iris, through which the **pupil** is seen.

pupillometer
A device that performs **pupillometry**.

pupillometry
Measurement of **pupil** diameter.

pure alexia
Perceptual disturbance causing complete inability to read. Often, individual letters can be identified, but they cannot be grouped. *Synonym is* ***alexia without agraphia***.

Purkinje blue arcs
Entoptic phenomenon causing the appearance of blue arcs radiating from the **fovea** towards the **optic nerve head** when a red light is presented in the nasal **macula** region. Due to excitation of neighbouring nerve fibres serving the **S-cones**. *Synonym is* ***blue arcs phenomenon***.

Purkinje images
Reflections caused by the changes in **refractive index** through the eye. Can be used to estimate **anterior chamber** depth. *Synonym is* ***Purkinje–Sanson images***.

Purkinje shift
The shift in peak wavelength sensitivity between **scotopic/photopic** conditions (~505 to 555 nm).

Purkinje tree
Synonym of ***angioscotoma***.

Purkinje–Sanson images
Synonym of ***Purkinje images***.

pursuit
Synonym of ***smooth pursuit***.

push down method
A gross test of **amplitude of accommodation**, useful for patients with learning difficulties. Start with the target too close to see, and move it back until first seen by the patient. Not as accurate as the **push up method**.

push up method
Method of assessing **amplitude of accommodation**. An accommodative target is presented at a level that the patient can comfortably see; the target is gradually moved towards the patient, and the patient is asked to report when they can no longer focus on the image.

PV-16
Abbreviation of ***precision vision 16***.

PVD
Acronym of ***posterior vitreous detachment****.*

Px
Acronym of patient.

PXE
Acronym of ***pseudoxanthoma elasticum****.*

PXF
Acronym of ***pseudoexfoliation syndrome****.*

PXM
Acronym of pseudoexfoliative material.

PXS
Acronym of ***pseudoexfoliation syndrome****.*

pyogenic
A bacterial infection that makes pus.

pyogenic granuloma
Benign **pedunculated** tumour that typically develops at a site of previous trauma or from a **chalazion**.

P

Q

q.d.
Acronym of quaque die (daily).

q.d.s.
Acronym of quater die sumendus (four times daily).

q.i.d.
Acronym of quater in die (four times daily).

q2h
Abbreviation of quaque 2 hora (every 2 hours, for example).

quadrantanopia
Visual field loss in the whole of one quadrant of the field.

quiescence
The state of a nerve cell when not acting (quiet).

Q

R

RAAB
Acronym of ***rapid assessment of avoidable blindness.***

random dot stereogram
An autostereogram containing no actual image at all, only a form perception that can be accessed by binocular processing of common dots. The Lang test is an example. *Synonym is* ***randot.***

randot
Synonym of ***random dot stereogram.***

RAP
Acronym of retinal angiomatous proliferation.

RAPD
Acronym of ***relative afferent pupillary defect.***

raphé
The horizontal equator of the **fundus**.

rapid assessment of avoidable blindness
A standardised survey methodology used to estimate the prevalence and main causes of avoidable blindness in over 50s of any given population. *Acronym is* ***RAAB.***

rapid assessment of refractive error
A standardised survey methodology used to estimate the prevalence of uncorrected refractive error in any given population. *Acronym is* ***RARE.***

rapid serial visual presentation
Method of presenting a series of images or (usually) words in a fixed **location** such that they can be processed more rapidly and without the need to make **saccade**s. *Acronym is* ***RSVP.***

RARE
Acronym of ***rapid assessment of refractive error.***

Rashbass stimulus
Synonym of ***step-ramp stimulus.***

rate of angular expansion
Used to judge the speed of movement through an **optic array** towards the **focus of expansion.**

Rayleigh criterion
The centre of one **Airy disc** must be separate from the first minimum of another to perceive two stimuli.

Rayleigh match
A colour match used in **anomaloscope**s to detect red-green defects.

Raynaud's syndrome
Poor peripheral body circulation – associated with **normotensive glaucoma** (poor blood flow causing nerve death).

RB
Acronym of ***Rose Bengal stain****.*

RBC
Acronym of red blood cell.

RD
Acronym of ***retinal detachment****.*

RE
Acronym of right eye.

reading addition
Synonym of ***addition****.*

real image magnification
Synonym of ***transverse magnification****.*

rebound nystagmus
Nystagmus caused by a return to the **primary position** following a prolonged period of time in eccentric **gaze**.

receptive field
An area in real space or on the retina from which a neuron can be affected. *Acronym is* ***RF****.*

receptor theory
For two separate stimuli to be perceived, a gap of one receptor must be present between their images on the retina.

recession
Weakening operation on **extraocular muscle**. Muscle is disinserted and reattached more posteriorly.

recovery point
The maximum amount of prism required such that **fusion** is restored after reaching the **break point**.

R

recumbent spectacles
Spectacles for use either lying down or whilst hunched over. Contain prisms in both eyes which move the image by up to 90°.

red-free filter
Makes red structures such as blood vessels appear blacker when used in an optical system.

Redmond Smith technique
Synonym of ***Smith's method****.*

reference electrode
Used in electrophysiology to quantify what part of a signal is noise; whatever is picked up by the reference electrode is subtracted from the active electrode value.

reflex accommodation
The automatic response to blur to maintain a clear retinal image.

reflex tears
Stimulated tears. ~100× greater production rate than **basal tears**.

refraction
The measurement of **vergence** of light. Often used to refer to the determination of a spectacle prescription by an **optometrist**.

refractive ametropia
Ametropia caused by the refractive component of the eye.

refractive index
Value that represents the amount of change in direction a medium will exert on light as it passes into it. *Acronym is* ***RI****. Synonym is* ***index of refraction****.*

R

refractive intraocular lens
An **intraocular lens** whose refractive power changes from the centre to the periphery. Gives good intermediate vision.

refractive lens exchange
Similar to **cataract** surgery – phakoemulsification and replacement with a new lens – but refers to the procedure when it is done as an alternative to laser surgery. *Acronym is* ***RLE****. Synonym is* ***clear lens exchange****.*

refractometry
A non-clinical tear film protein test; uses the fact that tear proteins have different **refractive index** to water.

Regan low contrast charts
A series of **logMAR** charts at different **contrast**s for children.

regression
A change back to the previous prescription following refractive surgery.

Reichardt detector
A model of motion detection involving two photoreceptors inputting to a single cortical neuron. A delay in the signal from the first photoreceptor enables detection of directional motion. *Synonym is **Hassenstein–Reichardt detector**.*

Reis–Bücklers' dystrophy
Anterior **corneal** dystrophy: early onset in life with **corneal erosions**. Honeycomb-like epithelium.

relative afferent pupillary defect
A difference in the amount of constriction between the **pupils** in response to light. Diagnosed with the **swinging flashlight test**. Indicates optic nerve pathology. *Acronym is **RAPD**. Synonyms are **afferent pupillary defect** and **Marcus Gunn pupil**.*

relative distance magnification
Magnification by bringing things closer. Most magnifiers work by this method.

relative hyperopic peripheral defocus
Describes the fact that most **minus lenses**, despite appropriately correcting **myopia** at the **fovea**, undercorrect at the peripheral retina. *Acronym is **RHPD**.*

relative luminous efficiency
The perceived lack of brightness in wavelengths at edge of the sensitivity range.

relative peripheral hyperopic defocus
The amount of refractive error at the peripheral retina, as compared to the refractive error at the fovea. It is believed that peripheral defocus may stimulate progression of **myopia**, even when foveal refraction is fully corrected.

relative scotoma
A **scotoma** that still has some sensitivity to bright stimuli.

relative size magnification
Magnification by making things larger.

relucency
The scattering of light by a heterogenous medium, making structures visible.

remote refraction
A method used in **tele-optometry** involving a remotely controlled **phoropter** and video conferencing system, allowing an **optometrist** to conduct a **refraction** without being physically present.

repetition priming
The fact that objects are more quickly recognised if they have been seen before.

R

representational unilateral neglect
A form of **unilateral neglect** in which attention for half of imagined or remembered images is impaired. Similar to **aphantasia**, but on one side only.

RER
Acronym of rough endoplasmic reticulum.

resection
Strengthening operation on **extraocular muscle**. Muscle is disinserted, a piece is removed, and the muscle is reinserted in the same place.

residual shell error
The dioptric distance between the far point sphere and **Petzval surface.**

Ret
Abbreviation of ***retinoscopy****.*

reticular drusen
A type of **drusen** usually found in the superotemporal **macula**. *Synonym is* ***reticular pseudodrusen****.*

reticular pseudodrusen
Synonym of ***reticular drusen****.*

retinal artery occlusion
Refers to either a **central retinal artery** occlusion or a branch retinal artery occlusion.

retinal break
Any full thickness defect of the neurosensory retina.

retinal correspondence
The relationship between points in each retina that correspond to the same visual direction.

R

retinal dehydrogenase
Converts **all-trans-retinal** to **all-trans-retinol**.

retinal densitometry
A method of measuring the rate of photopigment regeneration.

retinal detachment
Separation of the neurosensory layers of retina from the **retinal pigment epithelium**. May be a **tractional retinal detachment**, **serous retinal detachment**, or a **rhegmatogenous retinal detachment**. *Acronym is RD.*

retinal disparity
Synonym of ***fixation disparity****.*

retinal flow
Optic flow taking into account movement of the eyes and head to calculate real movement.

retinal ganglion cell
One of the cell types found in the retina; their cell bodies are located in the **ganglion cell layer**. *Synonyms are **gangliocyte** and **ganglion cell**.*

retinal migraine
*Synonym of **ocular migraine**.*

retinal pigment epithelium
Cuboidal monolayer (columnar at the **fovea**) pigmented with **melanosomes**, lying between the **choroid** and neurosensory retina. Pigmentation helps to prevent scatter of light within the eye. Phagocytoses photoreceptor outer segments. *Acronym is **RPE**.*

retinal slip
Movement of an image across the retina.

retinal tear
A break in the neurosensory retina, usually caused by traction. If left untreated (by laser), may progress to a **rhegmatogenous retinal detachment**.

retinal tuft
Projections of retinal tissue found at the **vitreous** base. Found in most of the population.

retinal vein occlusion
Occlusion of part (**branch retinal vein occlusion**) or all (**central retinal vein occlusion**) of the retinal vein. May be **ischaemic retinal vein occlusion, non-ischaemic retinal vein occlusion**, or papillophlebitis. May be caused by **arteriolosclerosis** and blood **dyscrasias**. May lead to **hundred day glaucoma**. *Acronym is **RVO**.*

retinitis pigmentosa
Rod-cone dystrophy (rods affected more than cones). Due to the **retinal pigment epithelium** phagocytosing photoreceptor outer segments too quickly. Causes **nyctalopia** and gradually restricting tunnel vision. Signs include **bone spicule pigmentation**, attenuated vessels, and **pallor** of the **optic nerve head**. *Acronym is **RP**.*

retinitis punctata albescens
A variant of **retinitis pigmentosa**, presents at less than 30 years of age. **Fundus** appearance is of scattered white dots, eventually developing **bone spicule pigmentation**.

retinoblastoma
Cancer of the photoreceptors. Occurs in young children (usually 3 months). Causes **leukocoria**.

retinogeniculocortical pathway
*Synonym of **geniculocortical pathway**.*

retinopathy
Any non-inflammatory damage to the retina.

retinopathy of prematurity
Condition caused by premature infants being exposed to very high levels of oxygen in incubators. This causes a relative **hypoxia** later on in early development, causing **neovascularisation** of the retina which can lead to haemorrhaging, scarring, traction, and **tractional retinal detachment**. *Acronym is **ROP**. Synonym is **retrolental fibroplasia**.*

retinoschisis
Splitting of the retina. Usually occurs at the **outer plexiform layer**; can also occur at the **inner nuclear layer**. More common in **hyperopes**.

retinoscope
The device used in **retinoscopy**.

retinoscopy
Objective measurement of the refractive error of an eye using a light reflected from the retina. *Abbreviation is **Ret**. Synonyms are **photoscopy**, **shadow test**, **skiametry**, and **skiascopy**.*

retinotectal pathway
The visual pathway in the brain that travels via the **superior colliculus** (10% of retinal **ganglion cells** lead here). *Synonym is **extrageniculostriate cortex**.*

retinotopic
Having a map of the retina (as in the **lateral geniculate nucleus** and **primary visual cortex**).

retrobulbar
Behind the **globe**(s).

retrobulbar neuritis
*Synonym of **retrobulbar optic neuritis**.*

R

retrobulbar optic neuritis
Inflammation of the optic nerve behind the **optic nerve head**. Causes **visual field** defects; occurs at ~20 years of age. Indicates multiple sclerosis. Fast recovery. *Synonym is **retrobulbar neuritis**.*

retrolental fibroplasia
*Synonym of **retinopathy of prematurity**.*

retrolental space of Erggelet
*Synonym of **Berger's postlenticular space**.*

reversible spectacles
Spectacles with one eye glazed for distance vision and one for near. A useful solution for **monocular** presbyopic patients, as both prescriptions are in one frame.

RF
*Acronym of **receptive field**.*

RGP
*Acronym of **rigid gas permeable**.*

rhabdomyosarcoma
A highly malignant tumour of striated muscle. Often occurs in children. May cause **strabismus**, **proptosis**, and reduced **ocular motility**.

rhegmatogenous retinal detachment
Retinal detachment caused by accumulation of fluid under a **retinal tear**. *Acronym is **RRD**.*

rheum
Mucus that accumulates and dries near the **lacrimal caruncle** during sleep.

rheumatoid spondylitis
*Synonym of **ankylosing spondylitis**.*

rhodopsin
The photopigment found in rods. *Synonym is **visual purple**.*

RHPD
*Acronym of **relative hyperopic peripheral defocus**.*

RI
*Acronym of **refractive index**.*

Ricco's area
Maximum area over which **Ricco's law of complete spatial summation** occurs.

Ricco's law of complete spatial summation
Luminance threshold multiplied by stimulus area is constant up to **Ricco's area**.

Riddoch phenomenon
Form of **blindsight** in which patients have **statokinetic dissociation** within a **visual field** defect. A type of **gnosanopsia**. *Synonyms are **attentional blindsight** and **Riddoch syndrome**.*

Riddoch syndrome
*Synonym of **Riddoch phenomenon**.*

Rieger anomaly
Posterior embryotoxon, **corectopia**, and iris **hypoplasia**. Associated with **buphthalmos**.

rigid gas permeable
A contact lens made of a hard material that allows the passage of oxygen through the lens. *Acronym is **RGP**. Synonyms are **corneal lens** and **gas permeable lens**.*

rigid hydrogel contact lens
A contact lens with a **rigid gas permeable** centre and hydrogel periphery. Only used in **keratoconus/cornea**l irregularities. Tend to break at the dividing line between the hard and soft lens.

riMLF
Acronym of ***rostral interstitial nucleus of the medial longitudinal fasciculus.***

ringing
A low-amplitude oscillation of the eyes that occurs normally during the onset of **smooth pursuit**.

Riolan muscle
Portion of the **orbicularis oculi** next to the **eyelid** margin.

RIR
Acronym of retinal ***illuminance*** *response.*

rivalry
The perception of a different stimulus by each eye, causing **confusion** and **mosaic rivalry**.

Rivermead behavioural inattention test
Synonym of ***behavioural inattention test.***

Rizzuti's sign
In **keratoconus**, a conical reflection seen on the nasal **cornea** when a light is shone from the other side.

RK
Acronym of radial keratotomy.

R

RLE
Acronym of ***refractive lens exchange.***

RNA
Acronym of ribonucleic acid.

RNFL
Acronym of retinal nerve fibre layer.

rod monochromatism
Condition in which no cones work at all. *Synonym is* ***complete monochromatism.***

rod-cone break
The point during **dark adaptation** at which rods become more sensitive than cones.

rodent ulcer
A noduloulcerative **basal cell carcinoma.**

roll
Tilting of the head left or right.

Rønne nasal step
Sign of **glaucoma** – step-like coalescence of **scotoma**s above and below the **raphé** in the nasal **visual field.** *Synonym is* ***nasal step.***

ROP
Acronym of ***retinopathy of prematurity.***

Rose Bengal stain
Stains damaged **cornea**l and **conjunctiva**l cells to identify damage to the eye. Stings on instillation. *Acronym is* ***RB.***

roseolae
Dilated iris capillaries in **iridocyclitis** in patients with **syphilis.**

rosette
A paper strip impregnated with **Rose Bengal stain.**

rostral
Anterior.

rostral interstitial nucleus of the medial longitudinal fasciculus
The vertical **saccade** control centre. Situated in the **mesencephalic reticular formation.** *Acronym is* ***riMLF.***

RP
Acronym of ***retinitis pigmentosa.***

RPE
Acronym of ***retinal pigment epithelium.***

RPM
Acronym of rapidly progressing myopia.

RRD
Acronym of ***rhegmatogenous retinal detachment.***

RSVP
Acronym of ***rapid serial visual presentation.***

RTA
Acronym of road traffic accident.

rubeosis iridis
Neovascularisation from the **pupil** margin across the iris as a response to **ischaemia**, for example in diabetes or an old **central retinal vein occlusion**.

rubeotic glaucoma
Glaucoma caused by blockage of the **trabecular meshwork** by **rubeosis iridis**.

Rubin vase
A perceptual illusion in which a vase also looks like a pair of faces in profile.

rubor
Redness.

RVI
Acronym of referral of vision impaired patient.

RVO
Acronym of ***retinal vein occlusion.***

Rx
Abbreviation of prescription.

R

S

s
Abbreviation of sans (without).

S-cone
Abbreviation of blue cone.

S/P
Acronym of specific precaution.

saccade
A ballistic eye movement from one point of **fixation** to another. The fastest type of eye movement known.

saccade initiation failure
Inability to change **fixation** using **saccades**. **Vestibulo-ocular reflex** remains intact. Usually only horizontal saccades are impaired, although vertical can also be affected. Patients thrust their head to put the eyes in an intended direction. *Synonyms are **Cogan's apraxia**, **ocular apraxia**, and **oculomotor apraxia**.*

saccadic dead time
The point in time after programming of a **saccade** after which new visual information will not affect the outcome of the saccade.

saccadic inhibition
Reduced likelihood of a **saccade** being executed in the 50–70 ms following a sudden change in visual stimulus.

saccadic intrusion
Small instabilities of **fixation**, larger than **microsaccades**, in which the eyes briefly move away from fixation. Two types are seen in normals: **square-wave intrusions** and **saccadic pulses**.

saccadic pulse
A type of **saccadic intrusion** often seen in normals in which the eyes are rapidly deviated away from the point of **fixation** followed immediately by a return to target. There are two types: **single saccadic pulse** and **double saccadic pulse**.

saccadic suppression
During a **saccade**, visual input is suppressed to prevent a blurred retinal image.

saccadomania
*Synonym of **opsoclonus**.*

saddle bridge
*Synonym of **comfort bridge**.*

SAFE
Ocular **motility test**ing demonstrated **smooth pursuit** that was Smooth, Accurate, and Fully Extensive.

sagittal plane
The anatomical plane that divides the body into two symmetrical halves. Also used to refer to this plane of a spectacle lens.

Saladin's 1:1 rule
Used to estimate prism required in **eso** deviations. The **recovery point** of the **negative fusional reserves** should be at least the same magnitude as the **esophoria**. If it is not, the prism required is half of the difference between these. For **exo** deviations, use **Sheard's criterion** or **Percival's criterion**.

saline
0.9% sodium chloride.

salmon patches
Large **dot haemorrhages/blot haemorrhages** are called this when seen in **non-proliferative sickle cell retinopathy**.

Salus' sign
Deflected veins at arteriovenous crossings in **hypertensive retinopathy**.

Salzmann nodular degeneration
Nodules of superficial stromal opacity. Occurs following **inflammation** (even if long ago).

SAO
*Acronym of **successive alternate occlusion**.*

S

SAP
Acronym of standard automated perimetry.

sarcoidosis
A rare systemic granulomatous disease, onset in 40s. A third of patients have ocular problems: **uveitis**/dry eye.

sarcoma
Cancer of connective tissue, muscle, or bone.

Sattler's layer
The innermost, smaller layer of the **choroid**al blood vessels.

Sattler's veil
Cloudy vision and haloes around light due to **corneal oedema**.

Sbisa bar
Similar to a **neutral density filter bar** but also contains a red filter which allows the image seen by the eye covered by the bar to be more easily appreciated. *Synonym is **Bagolini filter bar**.*

scalar Grassman's law
When both sides of a metameric match are altered by the same proportional amount (e.g. with filters), the match holds.

scanning laser polarimetry
Technique of using polarised light to measure **nerve fibre layer** thickness. The GDx is an example.

scanpath
The path taken by the eyes around a visual scene.

Scarpa's ganglion
The ganglion of the **vestibular nerve**.

SCC
*Acronym of **squamous cell carcinoma**.*

Scheerer's phenomenon
*Synonym of **blue field entoptic phenomenon**.*

Scheie classification
Grading scale for **hypertensive retinopathy**; grades **hypertension** and **arteriolosclerosis** separately.

Scheimpflug camera
Gives a lot of **depth of focus** to generate 3D images.

Schiøtz tonometry
Contact **tonometer** which measures pressure by applanating with a known weight.

Schirmer's tear flow test
Paper tabs inserted at the eyes nasally, left for 5 minutes. <10 mm wetting is abnormal and may indicate dry eye.

Schlemm's canal
Annular vessel that collects **aqueous humour** from the **channels of Sondermann**. *Synonym is **canal of Schlemm**.*

S

Schmidt's sign
In female **protan** defect carriers, there is a reduced sensitivity to long wavelengths.

Schnyder dystrophy
Anterior **corneal** dystrophy. Presents in patients between 10 and 20 years of age with visual symptoms. Sub-epithelial crystalline opacities.

Schwalbe's line
The exact point where the **cornea** becomes the **limbus** (end of **Descemet's membrane**). Viewed with a goniolens.

Schwann cell
Glial cell that myelinates nerve cells in the peripheral nervous system.

scissor reflex
Two reflex movements in different directions during **retinoscopy**. Suggests **keratoconus** or **cataracts**.

sclera
White protective layer covering most of the eye, except at the **cornea**. Contains collagen, proteoglycans, elastic fibres. Relatively **avascular**.

scleral buckle
Used to treat anterior **retinal detachments**. A silicone band is sewn onto the **sclera** at the site of the detachment to push the **retinal pigment epithelium** towards the retina.

scleral contact lens
A contact lens that covers a larger area than a standard contact lens, reducing pressure on the **cornea** and **limbus**. *Synonym is **haptic lens**.*

scleral depression
*Synonym of **scleral indentation**.*

scleral indentation
Pressure applied to the outside of the **globe** in order to view the anterior **fundus**. *Synonym is **scleral depression**.*

scleral search coil
An **eye tracking** technique that involves sitting within a magnetic coil whilst wearing a hard contact lens. Difficult to tolerate for >30 minutes but enables recording of **torsional** eye movements. *Synonym is **search coil**.*

scleral slits
Refractive surgery: radial slits made outside the **cornea** (on the **sclera**). The results are fairly unpredictable.

scleral spur
The rigid circular **scleral** projection which anchors the **ciliary muscle** and some of the **trabecular meshwork.**

scleral stroma
Tough middle layer of the **sclera.** Contains dense fibrous tissue and **fibroblasts.** Fibrils are less organised here than in the **corneal stroma** (hence less transparent).

scleritis
Serious **inflammation** of the **sclera**; often **photophobia**, redness, dull pain, vision loss. Gradual onset. Treated with steroids, or in extreme cases, immunosuppressive drugs.

sclerocornea
Rare condition in which the patient is born without a **cornea** – the **sclera** just continues over the area.

scleromalacia perforans
Non-inflammatory necrotising anterior **scleritis.**

sclerosis
Hardening (Greek).

sclerotic scatter
Slit-lamp technique used to illuminate any **corneal** opacities. With slit-lamp **illumination** at 60° from the viewing system, focus the decoupled lamp at the **limbus** to scatter light through the cornea by total internal reflection. Opacities may glow and cause light to fail to transmit across the whole cornea.

SCN
Acronym of ***suprachiasmatic nucleus.***

SCO
Acronym of sphero-cylindrical over-refraction.

scotogenic contact lens
A contact lens with a painted pupil and graduated border, used to alleviate central **diplopia** without eliminating peripheral vision.

scotoma
Part of the **visual field** where there is reduced sensitivity.

scotomata
Occasionally used as the plural of the word **scotoma.**

scotopic
Low **illumination** levels in which rods are responsive but cones are not.

S

scotopic threshold response
In **electroretinography**, the negative wave due to **amacrine cells** and **ganglion cells**. Only occurs when a dim flash is presented to a dark-adapted patient. *Acronym is **STR**.*

scotopic vision
Vision in low light conditions.

screen fatigue
Burning, itching, **asthenopia**, etc. associated with excessive visual display unit use. Also wrist, back, neck pain, etc.

screen reader
Assistive technology that reads the contents of a screen, incorporating both **text-to-speech** and descriptors of other elements shown on the screen.

SE
Acronym of side effect.

sea-fan neovascularisation
Occurs in **proliferative sickle cell retinopathy**. Blood vessels grow into the **vitreous humour** and wave around like a sea fan.

SEAL
*Acronym of **superior epithelial arcuate lesion**.*

search coil
*Synonym of **scleral search coil**.*

sebaceous gland
A gland that secretes **sebum**.

sebaceous gland carcinoma
Highly malignant tumour of the **sebaceous glands**. Mimics **blepharitis**. May produce yellow material. Usually on upper **eyelid**.

seborrhoeic blepharitis
Blepharitis due to excessive secretion by the **meibomian glands** and/or **Zeis glands**.

sebum
Oily **lipid** substance that limits evaporation and keeps tears from **eyelid** skin.

second cranial nerve
Optic nerve.

second focal length
The distance at which the origin of focus of light must lie such that emergent light from a positive lens is rendered parallel.

secondary deviation
The deviation caused in the unaffected eye by **Sherrington's law of reciprocal innervation** when fixating with the affected eye.

secondary eye fields
Synonym of ***supplemental eye fields.***

secondary headache
Any form of **headache** which occurs secondary to some underlying condition.

secondary hypertension
Hypertension caused by a renal or endocrine pathology, or (rarely) congenital coarctation of the aorta.

secondary Jones test
Cotton bud is placed in the nose, and **sodium fluorescein** is injected into the **canaliculus.** The transmission of dye onto the bud indicates **nasolacrimal duct** patency. *Synonym is* ***Jones II test.***

secondary microtropia
A **microtropia** that was originally a larger angle **strabismus**, and reduced somehow.

secondary pigment dispersion syndrome
Pigment dispersion syndrome due to a displaced **intraocular lens.**

secondary vitreous
The type of **vitreous humour** present at birth and during life; displaces the **primary vitreous** anteriorly during gestation.

see-saw nystagmus of Maddox
Nystagmus in which one eye elevates and **intort**s whilst the other depresses and **extort**s; this is reversed and repeated.

SEF
Acronym of ***supplemental eye fields.***

segment top position
Vertical distance from the top of a bifocal segment to the **datum line**. *Acronym is STP.*

Seidel scotoma
Synonym of ***arcuate scotoma.***

Seidel test
Sodium fluorescein is instilled onto the **cornea** and observed closely to see if clear **aqueous humour** leaks through the pool of fluorescein. If it does, this indicates a full thickness wound of the eye.

S

semi-automated kinetic perimetry
Electronic type of **perimetry** that can correct for reaction times. *Acronym is **SKP**.*

semicircular canal
In the inner ear, contains fluid which passes to the **ampullae**. There are three in each ear, each oriented in alignment with one of the pairs of **extraocular muscles**.

SEN
Acronym of special educational needs.

senile arcus
*Synonym of **arcus senilis**.*

senile hyposecretion
The natural reduction in tear secretion rate that occurs with age. *Synonym is **acquired primary lacrimal deficiency**.*

senile macular degeneration
*Synonym of **age-related macular degeneration**.*

senile miosis
The gradual **miosis** that naturally occurs with age.

sensitivity regulation
The fact that **increment threshold** is always a fixed percentage of background luminance.

sensory esotropia
Esotropia that develops due to reduced sensory input to one eye.

sensory fusion
The ability to perceive two images and interpret as one; the **cortical** superposition of the retinal images from both eyes such that **diplopia** and **confusion** do not occur.

sensory ocular dominance test
A +2.00 DS (or similar) over-correction is added to each eye's final prescription separately. The eye in which the patient tolerates over-correction more is the non-dominant eye.

sentinel vessel
Larger blood vessels; may indicate extra blood being used to supply a **melanoma**.

separation difficulty
*Synonym of **crowding effect**.*

septo-optic dysplasia
Congenital brain abnormality characterised by **optic nerve hypoplasia**, absence of the septum pellucidum, and hypopituitarism. *Synonym is **de Morsier syndrome**.*

septum
Divides something into two.

sequelae
Synonym of ***muscle sequelae****.*

sequential stereo camera
Two pictures taken separately so that they may be viewed together to provide a pseudo-3D image. The **stereobase** is not constant, however, and the **pupil** must re-dilate between flashes of the camera.

SER
Acronym of smooth endoplasmic reticulum.

serous
Producing or resembling serum (having a thin/watery constitution).

serous retinal detachment
Retinal detachment due to **exudation** of material into the **subretinal space**. *Acronym is SRD. Synonym is* ***exudative retinal detachment****.*

SES
Acronym of ***steady eye strategy****.*

sessile
Stationary.

sessile drop method
A method of measuring **wetting angle**: a drop of liquid is placed on the surface to be measured, and the tangent formed is taken as the measurement.

seventh cranial nerve
Synonym of ***facial nerve****.*

SF
Acronym of ***short-term fluctuation****.*

SG
Acronym of specific gravity.

shadow test
Synonym of ***retinoscopy****.*

Shafer's sign
Grey specks seen in the **vitreous humour** (floating pigment or red blood corpuscles). Sign of **retinal detachment**. *Synonym is* ***tobacco dust****.*

S

Shaffer grading
Grading system for **anterior chamber angle** closure, graded as 0, I, II, III, or IV. 0 = closed, IV = wide angle.

Sheard's criterion
Used to estimate prism required in **exo** deviations. **Fusional reserve**s should be at least double the demand. Prism required = ⅔(magnitude of deviation) – ⅓(fusional reserves). For **eso** deviations, use **Saladin's 1:1 rule** or **Percival's criterion**.

Sheedy disparometer
Equipment used to measure the angle of **fixation disparity** (as opposed to **associated phoria**, which is measured with a **Mallett unit**).

Sheridan–Gardiner test
A six-metre calibrated **visual acuity** test. A child matches the letters using a matching card.

Sherrington's law of reciprocal innervation
For each eye, antagonistic muscles receive equal but opposite innervation.

Shh
Acronym of ***Sonic hedgehog homologue.***

shield ulcer
Deposits of bacteria found on the **cornea** in **vernal keratoconjunctivitis**.

shingles
Reactivation of the **varicella-zoster virus** in later life. *Synonym is* ***herpes zoster.***

short ciliary nerves
Branch from the ciliary ganglion, pierce the back of the eye, and innervate the iris, **cornea**, and **ciliary body**.

short wavelength sensitive automated perimetry
Used to assess **increment threshold**s in **S-cone**s. Stimulus is blue on yellow; stimulates **konio cells**. *Acronym is* ***SWAP.***

S

short-range motion
Motion within a **receptive field**'s spatial and temporal limits. Compare with **long-range motion**.

short-term fluctuation
In **perimetry**, the standard deviation of the difference between the responses given for the same areas (a check of the reliability of the test). Measured in decibels. *Acronym is* ***SF.***

SI
Acronym of ***sight impaired.***

sickle cell retinopathy
Similar to **diabetic retinopathy**; plus retinal holes. Classified as **proliferative sickle cell retinopathy** or **non-proliferative sickle cell retinopathy**.

siderosis
Describes an iron foreign body. If trapped in the iris, causes it to become darker and can cause a secondary **glaucoma**.

Siegrist streaks
Linear pigmented flecks that follow **choroid**al vessels in **hypertensive choroidopathy**.

signal detection theory
States that a stimulus is perceived when the evidence for a stimulus exceeds the evidence for no stimulus. Supersedes **high threshold theory**.

SIK
Acronym of ***sterile infiltrative keratitis***.

silicon hydrogel
Contact lens material. Oxygen binds to silicone, allowing six times more oxygen to reach the **cornea** than in traditional HEMA materials.

silver wiring
In **arteriosclerosis**, **copper wiring** becomes more pronounced and eventually appears silver.

simple cell
Type of cell found in the **primary visual cortex** with **receptive field**s that detect oriented edges.

simple episcleritis
Synonym of ***diffuse episcleritis***.

simple hyperopic astigmatism
One line focus of the astigmatic cone is at the retina, the other is behind.

simple myopic astigmatism
One line focus of the astigmatic cone is at the retina, the other is in front.

simulated distance exotropia
A **distance exotropia** due to **fusional reserves**.

simultagnosia
Synonym of ***simultanagnosia***.

simultanagnosia
Inability to perceive more than one object at a time. *Synonym is* ***simultagnosia***.

S

simultaneous colour contrast
The colour of a target's surround affects the perceived colour of the target.

simultaneous contrast
The luminance of a target's surround affects the perceived lightness of the target.

simultaneous perception
The ability to perceive two separate images.

simultaneous stereo camera
Uses prisms to take two pictures simultaneously so that they may be viewed together to provide a pseudo-3D image. Useful for patients who are unable to sit still, as the pictures are taken in one shot.

simultaneous vision contact lens
Multi/bifocal contact lenses that don't rely on moving to use the different powers, i.e. concentric or diffractive designs. **Contrast sensitivity** is compromised due to light scatter.

single saccadic pulse
A **saccadic pulse** in which the return to target is a slow drift.

sinuous side
A wavy type of spectacle side – waves out from head.

sinus
Any bay or cavity.

siRNA
Acronym of small inhibitory ribonucleic acid.

SITA
Acronym of ***Swedish interactive threshold algorithm.***

six-figure system
System for numbering refractive materials. The first three digits are the **refractive index** (after the decimal point); the last three are the **Abbe value** without the decimal point.

sixth cranial nerve
Synonym of ***abducens nerve.***

size constancy
The ability of the visual system to perceive objects as the same size despite varying visual angle.

size lens
Synonym of ***iseikonic lens.***

Sjögren's syndrome
Keratoconjunctivitis sicca caused by complete failure of the lacrimal system. Most likely in arthritic elderly women.

skew deviation
Vertical **strabismus** caused by brainstem or cerebellar disease.

skiametry
Synonym of ***retinoscopy.***

skiascopy
Synonym of ***retinoscopy.***

SKP
Acronym of ***semi-automated kinetic perimetry.***

sl
Abbreviation of slight deviation.

slab off
Adding base up prism into a lens by removing material.

slab on
Inducing base down prism into a lens by tilting it during the moulding process.

SLE
Acronym of slit-lamp examination/systemic lupus erythematosus.

sleep miosis
The **miosis** that occurs during sleep.

SLK
Acronym of ***superior limbic keratoconjunctivitis.***

SLM
Acronym of slit-lamp microscopy.

Sloan letter
Any of the 10 letters (C, D, H, K, N, O, R, S, V, and Z) commonly used on distance **visual acuity** charts, drawn with uniform stroke width on a 5 × 5 grid.

slow fusion
Fusion that overcomes **diplopia** in ~2–3 minutes. Input is received from the output of the **fast fusion** mechanism.

S

slow oscillations
In **electroretinography**, the initial light peak and oscillations every 30 minutes thereafter, following the fast oscillation.

SLT
*Acronym of selective **LASER** trabeculoplasty.*

small metre angle
Monocular convergence **metre angle**.

smart glasses
Spectacles incorporating a computer, often as a **head-mounted display** for **augmented reality**.

smart plug
A **punctal** plug that shortens and widens within the **punctum**. *Synonym is **form fit plug**.*

SMILE
Acronym of small incision lenticule extraction.

smile stain
*Synonym of **inferior arcuate stain**.*

Smith's method
Method of estimating **anterior chamber** depth. A horizontal slit-lamp beam is shone on both the **cornea** and lens; the gap seen between the two is determined, Pythagoras' theorem is used to estimate the actual depth of the chamber at that point. *Synonym is **Redmond Smith technique**.*

smooth pursuit
A tracking eye movement in which the eyes move smoothly. *Synonym is **pursuit**.*

SMTF
*Acronym of **spatial modulation transfer function**.*

S

snail track degeneration
Peripheral retinal atrophy, more common in **myopia**. Similar to **lattice degeneration**, but milder.

Snellen fraction
A way of expressing **visual acuity**. (The distance a target is viewed)/(the distance at which the detail of the target would subtend one minute of arc at the retina).

Snellen letters
Letters constructed on a 5 × 5 grid.

Sno strips
A variation on **Schirmer's tear flow test**. Strips are placed temporally, patient looks up. Time taken to wet 1 cm is measured.

snow banking
A grey-white **plaque** of the inferior pars plana (hard to see without using **scleral indentation**).

snow blindness
Synonym of ***photokeratitis****.*

snowflake cataract
Cataract caused by hyperglycaemia drawing water into the lens by osmosis. Causes a myopic shift. Sign of diabetes. Reversible.

snowflake degeneration
Degeneration of the vitreous and peipheral retina, causing the appearance of crystalline intraretinal deposits. Symptoms include reduced **visual acuity** and **myodesopsia**. Risk of **retinal detachment**.

SNRI
Acronym of serotonin-norepinephrine reuptake inhibitor.

SNS
Acronym of somatic nervous system/sympathetic nervous system.

SO
Acronym of ***superior oblique****.*

sodium cromoglicate
An anti-inflammatory mast cell stabiliser.

sodium fluorescein
An orange ophthalmic dye that fluoresces green under short wavelength blue light. Used to assess the integrity of the **cornea**, the fit of contact lenses, and in **fluorescein angiography**. *Abbreviation is* ***NaFl****. Synonym is* ***fluorescein****.*

soft drusen
Larger than **hard drusen**, indistinct, often become confluent. *Synonym is* ***diffuse drusen****.*

soft exudates
Synonym of ***cotton wool spots****.*

Sonic hedgehog homologue
A gene that reduces the expression of the PAX6 gene; mutations in this can cause **cyclopia**, since PAX6 causes the development of two eyes. *Acronym is* ***Shh****.*

S

Sonksen–Silver test
A letter-matching test of **visual acuity**.

Sorsby's fundus dystrophy
Condition that typically presents in the 2nd–4th decades of life. Yellow **plaques**, **choroidal neovascularisation**, and atrophy, due to thickened **Bruch's membrane**.

SOTSS
Acronym of ***superior oblique tendon sheath syndrome****.*

sovereign top
In fused bifocals, a small lining of gold leaf (or other alloy) applied at the segment top to reduce reflections.

space eikenometer
A device that measures the extent of **aniseikonia**.

spasmus nutans
A form of **infantile onset nystagmus** accompanied by an **abnormal head posture** and involuntary head movements.

spatial antagonism
Synonym of ***lateral inhibition****.*

spatial disorientation
The inability to localise objects correctly.

spatial frequency
The number of cycles per degree of a stimulus.

spatial modulation transfer function
The relationship between **spatial frequency** and **contrast** threshold. Describes an optical system's transfer quality. *Acronym is SMTF.*

S

spatial tuning
The fact that **ganglion cell**s respond better to stimuli of a certain size (due to **lateral inhibition**).

SPE
Acronym of superficial punctate erosion.

spectacle blur
A reduction in **visual acuity** with spectacles following hard contact lens removal (usually PMMA) caused by **corneal** reshaping.

spectral domain optical coherence tomography
Type of space encoded **frequency domain optical coherence tomography**. The reflectivity at different wavelengths is analysed. *Synonym is* ***Fourier domain optical coherence tomography.***

speculum
Implement used to keep a patient's eye open during surgery.

SPEE
Acronym of superficial punctate epithelial erosion.

sph
Abbreviation of sphere.

sphenoid bone
Makes up the back of the **orbit**; holds the cranium together.

sphenoid sinuses
At the centre of the skull, in the **sphenoid bone**. One of the paranasal **sinuses**.

sphenoidal ridge meningioma
Tumour of the meninges that cross the **sphenoid bone** ridge. Causes **proptosis**.

sphere curve
Number that, when combined with the **base curve** of a lens, should equal the lens sphere power.

spherical manipulation
Modification of the spherical component of a spectacle prescription in order to drive **accommodation** to correct a **heterophoria** or **strabismus**. Calculated using the patient's **accommodative convergence:accommodation ratio**.

spheroidal degeneration
Amber opacities at the **limbus**. Due to hot, windy climate and ultraviolet light exposure. *Synonym is* ***climatic droplet keratopathy.***

spherule
The synaptic terminal of rod cells. Possesses a single synaptic cleft.

sphincter pupillae
Ring of smooth muscle fibres around the **pupil**. When it contracts, **miosis** occurs.

Spielmann occluder
A translucent occluder, used to perform the cover test whilst providing some view of the occluded eye.

splinter haemorrhage
Linear haemorrhage perpendicular to the **optic disc**. May indicate **glaucoma**. *Synonyms are* ***disc haemorrhage, Drance haemorrhage,*** *and* ***optic disc haemorrhage.***

spontaneous consecutive esotropia
A **consecutive esotropia** occurring in the absence of **extraocular muscle** surgery.

spontaneous consecutive exotropia
A **consecutive exotropia** occurring in the absence of **extraocular muscle** surgery.

spontaneous venous pulsation
Visible pulsation of retinal veins. *Acronym is* ***SVP.***

spot reading
Describes occasional reading for short periods of time, e.g. reading the back of packets (rather than books).

squamous
Describes a layered epithelium that consists, at least in its outer layer, of small scale-like cells.

squamous cell carcinoma
Skin cancer, commonly malignant. Rare cause of **blepharitis**. Can occur on the **conjunctiva**; looks like a **papilloma**. *Acronym is* ***SCC.***

square root law
Synonym of ***de Vries–Rose law.***

square-wave intrusion
A type of **saccadic intrusion** commonly seen in normal patients. There are two types: **monophasic square-wave intrusions** and **biphasic square-wave intrusions**. *Synonyms are* ***gegenrücke*** *and* ***square-wave jerk.***

square-wave jerk
Synonym of ***square-wave intrusion.***

S

SQUID
Acronym of superconductive quantum interference device.

squint
Synonym of ***strabismus.***

SR
Acronym of ***superior rectus.***

SRD
Acronym of ***serous retinal detachment.***

SRF
Acronym of ***subretinal fluid.***

SRNVM
Acronym of ***subretinal neovascular membrane.***

SSI
Acronym of severely sight impaired.

ST
Acronym of sight test.

staircase method
Psychophysical method in which stimulus intensity is increased until perceived, then reduced by a lesser amount until not perceived, then increasing by a smaller amount again, etc., until exact threshold is found.

staphylococcal blepharitis
Blepharitis due to **staphylococcus** infection.

staphylococcus
Synonym of ***staphylococcus aureus.***

staphylococcus aureus
A **Gram-positive** bacteria; 55% of all eye infections are believed to be caused by this. *Synonym is* ***staphylococcus.***

staphyloma
A black protrusion of the **uvea** poking through a weak structure anywhere in the eye. Could be peripapillary, posterior, etc.

stare optokinetic nystagmus
Optokinetic nystagmus in which the viewer attempts to maintain fixation, despite a moving visual scene. Slow phases are shorter than in **look optokinetic nystagmus**.

Stargardt disease
Inherited disease affecting the **retinal pigment epithelium** and **macula** in patients under 20 years old. Causes **bull's eye maculopathy, hard drusen**, and reduced **visual acuity**. *Acronym is STGD. Synonym is* ***juvenile macular degeneration.***

static perimetry
Perimetry in which the stimulus is in a fixed position but is presented at different levels of brightness.

statokinetic dissociation
The ability to perceive motion without form. In patients with **blindsight**, this is known as **Riddoch phenomenon**. *Synonym is* ***astatikopsia.***

steady eye strategy
Technique for reading by **eccentric viewing** in visually impaired patients. View with the **preferred retinal locus** and move the page, keeping the eyes still. *Acronym is **SES**.*

steady state electroretinography
The case in **electroretinography** in which the flashes presented are fast enough that a sine wave is seen on the result: photoreceptors are responding slowly.

Steele–Richardson–Olszewski syndrome
*Synonym of **progressive supranuclear palsy**.*

Stellwag's sign
Lagophthalmos associated with **Graves' disease**.

stem cell
An undifferentiated cell made in the bone marrow.

stenopaeic disc
A small slit that can be introduced in a trial frame to find the **axis** of **astigmatism** of a patient. *Synonym is **stenopaeic slit**.*

stenopaeic slit
*Synonym of **stenopaeic disc**.*

stenosis
An abnormal narrowing of a blood vessel (or any other tubular structure).

step-ramp stimulus
Smooth pursuit testing paradigm in which the tracking target jumps away from fixation, then moves constantly back towards (and beyond) the initial fixation point. *Synonym is **Rashbass stimulus**.*

stereoacuity
Describes the degree of depth perception of an individual or test.

S

stereoacuity threshold
The minimum angle of acuity at which **stereopsis** cannot be achieved (i.e. far away objects).

stereobase
The separation between two images used to create a 3D image.

stereopsis
The perception of three dimensions due to binocularity. The highest level of binocular vision.

sterile corneal infiltrate
A **corneal infiltrate** with a non-infective cause, such as those seen in **contact lens induced acute red eye** and **contact lens induced peripheral ulcers**.

sterile infiltrative keratitis
Keratitis characterised by mild pain, intact epithelium, mild **corneal** suppuration, mild **anterior chamber** reaction, peripheral corneal **lesions** <1 mm in size. *Acronym is **SIK**. Synonyms are **aseptic keratitis** and **sterile keratitis**.*

sterile keratitis
*Synonym of **sterile infiltrative keratitis**.*

STGD
*Acronym of **Stargardt disease**.*

Stickler syndrome
Developmental collagen disorder that causes high **myopia**, and can lead to **retinal detachment**, **cataract**, and **glaucoma**.

Stiles–Crawford effect
Cones all point towards the **pupil**; therefore light hitting them perpendicularly (on **axis**) gives a greater response. This helps to reduce the effect of light scatter within the eye.

Still's disease
*Synonym of **juvenile idiopathic arthritis**.*

Stilling–Türk syndrome
*Synonym of **Duane's retraction syndrome**.*

Stilling's canal
*Synonym of **hyaloid artery**.*

stimulus deprivation amblyopia
Amblyopia as a result of reduced visual input to one eye.

stimulus equivalence
In visual perception, the fact that we group objects together as the same type despite varying appearance of different objects within that group, e.g. all dogs are recognised as dogs and all tables are considered tables despite a wide variety of appearances.

stochastic resonance
The phenomenon by which a subthreshold stimulus may be detected due to noise boosting the signal, e.g. **intrinsic light**.

STP
*Acronym of **segment top position**.*

STR
*Acronym of **scotopic threshold response**.*

S

strabismic amblyopia
Amblyopia as a result of an adaptation to **confusion** due to **strabismus**.

strabismus
Manifest deviation in the angle between the eyes. *Synonyms are **heterotropia**, **squint**, and **tropia**.*

strabismus fixus
A bilateral **squint** in a fixed position, i.e. the eye won't leave that position. Usually there is an **abnormal head posture**. No **fusion**.

straight end
A spectacle side type that wraps around the head.

stratified
Layered.

strawberry naevus
*Synonym of **capillary haemangioma**.*

Strehl ratio
A measure of the quality of an optical system; the comparison of the point spread function of a diffraction limited wavefront to the aberrated wavefront.

striate cortex
*Synonym of **primary visual cortex**.*

stripe
In **V2**, refers to both **thick stripe**s and **thin stripe**s, but not **interstripe**s.

stroke
Loss of cerebral blood supply.

structural model theory
Theory that we recognise objects by looking at how the components fit together.

Sturge–Weber syndrome
Increased **episcleral** venous pressure, usually **buphthalmos**, possible **angle closure glaucoma**. Occurs in conjunction with a port-wine stain across the involved eye's side of face. *Synonym is **encephalotrigeminal angiomatosis**.*

Sturm's conoid
The bundle of rays in an astigmatic **pencil** between the two perpendicular line foci.

stye
*Synonym of **external hordeolum**.*

subarachnoid haemorrhage
Haemorrhage beneath the **arachnoid**, due to an alteration in intracranial pressure. This causes a sudden headache, followed by persistent headache. Pain worse on coughing.

subconjunctival haemorrhage
Bleeding beneath the **conjunctiva**. Patients often present with an alarmingly deep-red patch plainly visible externally, but no pain. Can be a sign of **hypertension**.

subepithelial melanosis
Oculodermal melanosis restricted to the ocular tissues. *Synonyms are* ***melanosis oculi*** *and* ***ocular melanocytosis***.

subjective fronto-parallel plane
Perceived plane in front of and parallel to the eyes (in anisometropes tilts towards the most myopic/least hyperopic eye). *Synonym is* ***empirical horopter***.

subjective relative afferent pupillary defect
Sign in which a light appears to be a different brightness when shone in each eye.

subluxation
Synonym of ***lens subluxation***.

subretinal fluid
Fluid found between the photoreceptors and **retinal pigment epithelium**, often as a result of **wet age-related macular degeneration**. *Acronym is SRF.*

subretinal neovascular membrane
Synonym of ***choroidal neovascular membrane***.

subretinal space
The potential space between the retina and **retinal pigment epithelium**.

substantia propria
Synonym of ***corneal stroma***.

subtractive colour production
Production of colour by starting with a single source of white light and using with filters to remove colours.

successive alternate occlusion
Technique used in **refraction** to check if a prescription is binocularly balanced: blur both eyes by the same amount; offer +0.25 DS to each; see if there is a discrepancy in the perceived vision **monocular**ly. *Acronym is* ***SAO***.

successive colour contrast
The effect of colour afterimage on the appearance of newly viewed colours.

S

sulcus
An inward dip of the brain (opposite of **gyrus**). Not as deep as a fissure. Plural is 'sulci'.

sunflower cataract
Cataract found in **Wilson's disease**.

sunrise syndrome
Describes an **intraocular lens** that has dislocated upward so that the lower edge of the lens is in the visual axis.

sunset syndrome
Describes an **intraocular lens** that has dislocated downward, so that the upper edge of the lens is in the visual axis.

superior colliculus
Part of the midbrain involved in visual processing and eye movements. *Synonyms are **optic tectum** and **tectum**.*

superior epithelial arcuate lesion
Mild **lesion** on the **cornea** due to mechanical pressure from a contact lens. *Acronym is **SEAL**.*

superior frontal eye fields
Part of the **frontal eye fields** involved in planning and initiating voluntary **saccade**s and **smooth pursuit** as well as maintaining **fixation** and smooth pursuit.

superior limbic keratoconjunctivitis
*Synonym of **contact lens induced superior limbic keratoconjunctivitis**.*

superior oblique
One of the six **extraocular muscle**s. Originates at the **annulus of Zinn**, passes through the **trochlea**, and inserts at the supero-temporal **globe**. Contraction causes **intorsion** (primarily), with **depression** and **abduction**. Innervated by the **contralateral trochlear nerve**. *Acronym is **SO**.*

superior oblique myokymia
Causes **oscillopsia** and **diplopia**. May be induced by depressing eyes. Cause unknown.

superior oblique tendon sheath syndrome
*Synonym of **Brown's syndrome**.*

superior rectus
One of the six **extraocular muscles**. Originates at the **annulus of Zinn** and inserts at the supero-nasal **globe**. Contraction causes **elevation** (primarily), with **intorsion** and **adduction**. Innervated by the **contralateral oculomotor nerve**. *Acronym is **SR**.*

supine
Lying down, face up.

supplemental eye fields
One of the **cortical eye fields**. Involved in generating **saccade**s using complex memorised behaviours. *Acronym is SEF. Synonym is* ***secondary eye fields***.

supplementary screen
A filter screen placed over a visual display unit to reduce glare and improve comfort.

support cane
A long cane that also provides support for the user.

suppression
An **adaptation** by the brain that eliminates perception of an aspect of vision; for example, areas of the vision in one eye may be suppressed in the case of misalignment of the eyes in order to prevent **diplopia** and **confusion**.

suppression scotoma
An area of the **visual field** in which vision is suppressed during binocular viewing.

suppurative keratitis
Synonym of ***microbial infiltrative keratitis***.

suprachiasmatic nucleus
The **optic tract** leads to this; involved in circadian rhythm. *Acronym is SCN.*

supraciliary space
The space between the **ciliary body** and **sclera**.

supraduction
Monocular **elevation**. *Synonym is* ***sursumduction***.

supranuclear gaze palsy
Describes an eye movement disorder due to a **lesion** prior to the nuclei of the **oculomotor nerve**, **abducens nerve**, or **trochlear nerve**, i.e. at the frontal cortex, **occipital cortex**, or the **gaze** centres.

supraorbital
Above the **orbit**.

suprathreshold perimetry
Perimetry done at a level expected to be seen easily in order to speed up the process. Not as accurate as threshold perimetry.

supraversion
Looking up with both eyes.

surgeon's spectacles
Spectacles with **Galilean telescope**s attached to the frame. Similar to some **low vision aids** in design.

sursumduction
*Synonym of **supraduction**.*

suspensory ligaments
*Synonym of **zonules of Zinn**.*

SVP
*Acronym of **spontaneous venous pulsation**.*

SWAP
*Acronym of **short wavelength sensitive automated perimetry**.*

Swedish interactive threshold algorithm
The algorithm used by the **Humphrey field analyser**; estimates response for a smooth curve. *Acronym is **SITA**.*

sweep visual evoked potential
Visual evoked potential in which the **spatial frequency** of a grating increased until the response waveform becomes flat. Used to estimate the **contrast sensitivity function**.

swept source optical coherence tomography
Type of time-encoded **frequency domain optical coherence tomography**. Received wavelengths are compared to emitted wavelengths. Penetrates deep through retina.

swinging flashlight test
Light is shone into alternating eyes to test for a **relative afferent pupillary defect**. If positive, there is a reduced direct response in the affected eye but normal consensual and near reflexes. *Synonym is **Marcus Gunn test**.*

swinging room experiment
Experiment that shows that we use visual cues to maintain balance: a child stands in a room, the wall swings away on a hinge, the child perceives this as losing their balance and overcompensates, causing them to fall over (or an adult standing in unfamiliar position).

Sx
Abbreviation of symptoms.

symblepharon
Adhesion of the **tarsal conjunctiva** to the **bulbar conjunctiva**.

symbol cane
A cane a blind person can use on rare occasions where they require assistance but which is usually kept hidden.

symmetrical convergence
Convergence in which both eyes converge by the same amount.

synaesthesia
Condition in which sensory stimulation also elicits perceptual experience in a different sensory modality, e.g. patients might 'see' sounds. Estimated prevalence of 4.4%.

synchysis scintallins
Liquified **vitreous humour** with cholesterol crystals that move when the eye does. There are rarely symptoms, and it is rarely a problem.

synechia
Adhesion of the iris to either the **cornea** (**anterior synechia**) or lens (**posterior synechia**). *Plural is **synechiae**.*

synechiae
*Plural of **synechia**.*

synergistic combination
The use of multiple drugs to achieve an end.

synoptophore
A type of **major amblyoscope**.

syphilis
A sexually transmitted infection that causes **madarosis**, **conjunctival** ulcers, **iridocyclitis** (with **roseolae**), **Argyll Robertson pupil**, **papilloedema**, **oculomotor nerve** palsy, **abducens nerve** palsy.

S

T

t.i.d.
Acronym of ter in die (thrice daily).

tachistoscopic
Describes an image that is presented for a very brief duration.

tachycardia
Rapid heart beating.

tachyphylaxis
Reduced response to a drug after the initial dose.

TAFC
Acronym of ***two alternative forced choice method****.*

tamoxifen
An anti-breast cancer drug. Side effects may include **corneal** deposits and **tamoxifen retinopathy**.

tamoxifen retinopathy
Crystalline deposits found between the **ganglion cell layer** and **inner plexiform layer** as a result of **tamoxifen** use. May cause a reduction in **visual acuity**.

tamponade
Pressing against something (in the eye this means **pneumatic retinopexy**).

tangent screen
Method of measuring **visual fields**. Black cloth hung on the wall; patient sits facing the wall with one eye occluded. Practitioner brings a target on a stick in from the edge, patient reports when seen. Repeated to elicit full visual fields. Very old fashioned and inaccurate by today's standards. *Synonym is* ***Bjerrum screen****.*

tarsal conjunctiva
The part of **conjunctiva** covering the inside of the **eyelids**. *Synonym is* ***palpebral conjunctiva****.*

tarsal gland
Synonym of ***meibomian gland****.*

tarsal muscles
Synonym of ***Müller's muscles****.*

tarsal plate
Dense elongated connective tissue that gives form and support to the **palpebrae**. *Synonym is* ***tarsus****.*

tarsus
Synonym of ***tarsal plate****.*

tarsus inferior
Lower **tarsal plate**. ~29 × 5 mm.

tarsus superior
Upper **tarsal plate**. ~29 × 10 mm.

Tc-cell
Abbreviation of cytotoxic T-cell.

TCA
Acronym of tricyclic antidepressant.

TCU test
Abbreviation of the City University test.

Td
Abbreviation of ***troland****.*

TD
Acronym of total diameter.

tear breakup time
Measure of the length of time the eye can be kept open without the tear film rupturing. *Acronym is* ***BUT****.*

tear duct
Synonym of ***nasolacrimal duct****.*

tear ferning
Tear test in which the tears are dried and electrolyte crystals examined.

tear lens
Tears trapped between a **rigid gas permeable** and the **cornea**. These tears act as a lens, contributing to the refractive correction provided by the contact lens.

tear prism
Raised line of tears found at the inferior **fornix**, held in place by liquid tension. In most individuals, this measures 0.2–0.4 mm in depth at the central **eyelid**, and 0.1–0.2 mm at the **canthi**.

Tecnis
A type of **diffractive intraocular lens** with concentric **Fresnel lens**es.

tectum
*Synonym of **superior colliculus**.*

TED
*Acronym of **thyroid eye disease**.*

TEF
Acronym of temporal eye fields.

teichopsia
A type of **hallucination** causing perception of zig-zag lines or 'castle battlement' shapes. A common form of **migraine aura**. *Synonym is **fortification spectra**.*

telangiectasia
Irregularly dilated and tortuous vessels.

tele-optometry
The provision of optometric services without the physical presence of an **optometrist**. Measurements and images may be recorded by a technician using appropriate tools. The results may be interpreted live by an optometrist (with discussion via video conferencing) or may be stored for later review.

telecanthus
Condition in which the medial **canthi** are temporally displaced (distance between eyes is normal).

teleopsia
Perceptual distortion causing objects to appear further away than they are. *Opposite is **pelopsia**.*

telescopic magnification
Magnification achieved by changing the subtended angle of the image. *Synonym is **angular magnification**.*

Teller acuity cards
Preferential looking test; targets are two gratings at either end of a card. Test at 38 cm. Practitioner must get to peephole in the centre of the card quickly to decide on response of patient.

temporal arteritis
*Synonym of **giant cell arteritis**.*

temporal contrast sensitivity function
A measure of how **contrast sensitivity function** varies with temporal resolution; the relationship describing how often flashes of an image must be presented to be seen at varying **contrasts**. *Synonym is **temporal modulation transfer function**.*

temporal crescent
*Synonym of **myopic crescent**.*

temporal frequency
Rate of change of stimulus (e.g. flicker) over time.

temporal impulse response function
Psychophysical descriptor of **temporal summation**; describes how likely a stimulus is to be perceived at all when it is flashed twice with various sized temporal gaps between presentations.

temporal modulation transfer function
*Synonym of **temporal contrast sensitivity function**.*

temporal retinal disparity
*Synonym of **crossed retinal disparity**.*

temporal summation
The phenomenon in the visual system that causes a light that is flashed twice with a very short gap in time between presentations to be perceived as a single flash.

temporary plug
A **punctum** plug designed for use as a trial before a permanent plug is inserted. Synthetic or made of collagen.

Tenon's capsule
Connective tissue sheet. Separates the eye from the orbital fat, and covers the **extraocular muscles** posterior to their insertions. *Synonyms are **bulbar sheath, facial sheath of the eye,** and **fascia bulbi**.*

tenotomy
The division of a tendon. Anterior tenotomy is a procedure sometimes used to reduce the **nystagmus amplitude**. Horizontal **extraocular muscles** are detached and reattached in their original location. The exact mechanism by which this works is unknown.

tensilon
A drug that causes improvement in **myasthenia gravis** for ~5 minutes.

tensilon test
Hess screen plot made, **tensilon** injected, Hess plotted again. If an improvement is seen on the second Hess plot, suggests **myasthenia gravis**.

T

teratogenic agent
Anything that can be done during pregnancy that could lead to congenital malformation.

teratology
Study of congenital malformation.

teratoma
A tumour resembling the germ layers of an embryo, possibly developing into organs or limbs.

terrestrial telescope
A **Keplerian telescope** with an erector prism or mirror system. Much longer as a result.

Terrien's marginal degeneration
Peripheral **corneal ectasia**, with steep 'shelf-like' drop-off. Usually appears in the superior **cornea**, often bilateral. Etiology unknown. May cause **astigmatism**.

Terror Subterra
A visual illusion, showing a monster chasing another monster down a tunnel. Due to the presence of the tunnel, one monster looks larger than the other but in fact the images are the same size.

tesselated fundus
The normal polygonal pigment appearance of a deeply pigmented **choroid**, especially in the periphery. *Synonyms are* ***fundus tigre***, ***leopard fundus***, ***mosaic fundus***, *and* ***tigroid fundus***.

tessellopsia
Geometric visual **hallucination** causing the perception of repeating patterns.

tetanus
Prolonged muscle contraction.

tetracaine
An **ester-linked anaesthetic**, routinely used by **optometrists**. Typically available at 0.5% concentration. *Synonym is* ***amethocaine***.

T

tetrachromatism
The presence of four photoreceptor types and the ability to use all four types.

Tetraflex
A type of accommodative **intraocular lens**. The lens moves, producing pseudo **accommodation**.

text-to-speech
Conversion of text from a computer (which may be acquired via **optical character recognition**) into speech as an **assistive technology**. *Acronym is* ***TTS***.

texton
In visual perception theory, the local features used for grouping of objects in pre-attentive vision.

TG
Acronym of glass transition temperature.

TGFB
Acronym of transforming growth factor beta.

Th-cell
Abbreviation of helper T-cell.

Thatcher illusion
Visual illusion in which an image of a human face is viewed upside-down, with the exception of the eyes and mouth, which are not inverted. It is difficult to notice that some features are inverted unless the rest of the face is viewed at its original orientation.

thick stripe
In **V2**, part of the **magnocellular pathway**. Sensitive to disparity, orientation, and movement.

thimerosal
An antiseptic. Limbal hyperaemia is sometimes a reaction to this. An ingredient formerly used in some contact lens products. *Synonym is **thiomersal**.*

thimerosal keratopathy
*Synonym of **contact lens induced superior limbic keratoconjunctivitis**.*

thin stripe
In **V2**, part of the **parvocellular pathway**. Colour coded.

thiomersal
*Synonym of **thimerosal**.*

third cranial nerve
*Synonym of **oculomotor nerve**.*

third visual pathway
A visual pathway, distinct from the **ventral stream** and partially overlapping with the **dorsal stream**. Passes through **hMT+** and mediates dynamic social cues.

Thorington card
A card used in the **modified Thorington test**, with a hole in the centre and both horizontal and vertical scales, used to indicate the magnitude of a **heterophoria**. Distance and near versions are available.

T

thrombocytopenia
Low platelet count. A complication of **leukaemia**. *Synonym is* ***Kasabach–Merritt syndrome****.*

thrombosis
A clot within a blood vessel.

thrombospondin
A protein with the ability to inhibit **angiogenesis**.

thrombus
Blood clot.

thrush
Synonym of ***candidiasis****.*

THS
Acronym of ***Tolosa–Hunt syndrome****.*

Thygeson's keratitis
Synonym of ***Thygeson's superficial punctate keratopathy****.*

Thygeson's superficial punctate keratopathy
Idiopathic epithelial **keratitis** presenting with small grey punctate dots. Symptoms include **photophobia**, dry eye, and foreign body sensation. *Synonym is* ***Thygeson's keratitis****.*

thymus
Organ in the upper anterior chest cavity. Lymphoid cells are matured here.

thyroid eye disease
Proptosis due to fluid in the **extraocular muscle**s. **Globe** stretching puts strain on the **optic nerve head** (**glaucoma** risk). Causes **chemosis**, lid retraction, inflammation of the **lacrimal caruncle**, **von Graefe sign**, and **Braley's sign**. Can occur without **hyperthyroidism**. Restricted **motility**. The muscles affected are typically (in order) the **inferior rectus**, **medial rectus**, **superior rectus**, and (occasionally) the **lateral rectus**. *Acronym is* ***TED****. Synonyms are* ***Graves' ophthalmopathy*** *and* ***Graves' orbitopathy****.*

TIA
Acronym of ***transient ischaemic attack****.*

TIB
Acronym of ***Turville infinity balance****.*

tight lens syndrome
Synonym of ***contact lens induced acute red eye****.*

tigroid fundus
Synonym of ***tesselated fundus****.*

tilted disc
The case in which the optic nerve enters the **orbit** at an oblique angle.

tilted room experiment
Experiment in which a runner runs on a treadmill, and the room is tilted. Runner adjusts tilt of body to compensate.

time domain optical coherence tomography
Commercial standard of **optical coherence tomography**: reference mirror moved over time; slow; 3D not practical.

Titmus fly test
*Synonym of **Titmus test**.*

Titmus test
Stereoacuity test using polarised spectacles. Patient views a large housefly which should appear in 3D if the patient has **stereopsis**. There are a few tests on the facing page which can give an indication of depth of stereopsis. *Synonyms are **Titmus fly test and Wirt test**.*

TLS
*Acronym of **tight lens syndrome**.*

Tm
*Acronym of **trabecular meshwork**.*

TNF
*Acronym of **tumour necrosis factor**.*

TNO test
Random dot stereograms made of red/green portions. Red/green glasses are worn by the patient to dissociate the eyes. A common test of **stereopsis**.

TO-1
*Synonym of **visual area middle temporal**.*

TO-2
*Synonym of **visual area medial superior temporal**.*

tobacco dust
*Synonym of **Shafer's sign**.*

Todd's syndrome
*Synonym of **Alice in Wonderland syndrome**.*

Tolosa–Hunt syndrome
A possible cause of **palsy** of the **oculomotor nerve**. *Acronym is **THS**.*

T

tonic accommodation
The amount of **accommodation** present when resting – in the dark, without a stimulus.

tonic cells
Synonym of ***parvo cells****.*

tonic convergence
The natural level of **convergence** caused by the presence of the **extraocular muscles**.

tonic innervation
The steady firing rate required to maintain an eye position. Firing rate is directly proportional to eccentricity of the eye position.

tonic pupil
Synonym of ***Adie's pupil****.*

tonicity
Comparison of solute concentration in relation to another solution.

Tono-Pen
A type of small portable contact **tonometer**.

tonometer
Any device that measures **intraocular pressure**.

tonometry
Measurement of **intraocular pressure**.

top-down processing
Model(s) of visual processing that assume a higher knowledge of the world is more important than its component parts.

topical
Administered outside of body.

T

topographagnosia
Topographical disorientation caused by damage to the **parahippocampal place area**. Loss of visual memory results in patients getting lost.

topographical disorientation
Condition in which patients get lost in familiar surroundings.

torsion
Either **intorsion** or **extorsion**; an eye movement in which the eye rotates about the visual axis.

total deviation map
On a **perimetry** printout, the left difference diagram. Analyses the height of the **visual field** as compared to age-normative data.

total dissociation
Describes a complete lack of 'common ground' for the eyes to focus on in the **visual field**, i.e. there is no stimulus for **fusion**.

total occlusion
Exclusion of form by patching. May also exclude light (if directly over the eye).

total penalisation
Amblyopia therapy in which the better eye is given a very strong lens (usually positive, but sometimes negative) to encourage use of the poor eye.

toxic amblyopia
Amblyopia caused by **lesion** or some other damage, e.g. tobacco or alcohol. *Synonym is **organic amblyopia**.*

toxic headache
Deep dull occipital pain. Increased pain with movement. Due to intoxication/hangover.

toxocara
A parasitic roundworm. Found in 80% of puppies (faeces). Causes **leukocoria** and blindness.

toxocariasis
Infection by **toxocara**.

toxoplasma
A parasitic worm found in cats.

toxoplasmosis
Infection by **toxoplasma**.

trabecular meshwork
Tissue between **Schlemm's canal** and **anterior chamber angle**. Provides a drainage route for **aqueous humour**. *Acronym is **Tm**.*

trabeculectomy
Flap opened in **sclera** to access **anterior chamber.** Piece of the **trabecular meshwork** is then removed. *Synonyms are **filtering operation** and **filtration surgery**.*

trachoma
Chlamydial conjunctivitis, causing scarring, causing **entropion**, causing **trichiasis,** causing **corneal oedema**, causing **neovascularisation**, causing blindness.

T

tractional retinal detachment
Retinal detachment due to a fibrous membrane on the retinal surface. *Acronym is **TRD**.*

trade magnification
The fact that many commercially available magnifiers are advertised as having 1× more magnification than just the power divided by 4; i.e. assumes that simply bringing the object into focus at 25 cm is 2× magnification.

transducin
Heterotrimeric G-protein. Converted to alpha-transducin and beta-gamma-transducin by metarhodopsin II.

transient ischaemic attack
Change in cerebral blood flow causing symptoms of **stroke** that persist less than 24 hours. *Acronym is **TIA**.*

transient visual evoked potential
Visual evoked potential elicited when sufficient time is given between stimuli presentation for the brain to return to rest.

transillumination
Condition in which the iris allows light to pass through, due for example to albinism or atrophy.

translating contact lens
A bifocal contact lens that relies on eye movement for the **addition** segment to displace to the centre of the **pupil**. Usually in hard lenses. *Synonyms are **alternating contact lens, alternating vision contact lens,** and **translating vision contact lens**.*

translating vision contact lens
*Synonym of **translating contact lens**.*

translocation
Swapping of parts of chromosomes.

transposons
Regions of chromosomes with no known function.

transpupillary thermotherapy
Intervention that uses a laser to apply heat to the **retinal pigment epithelium** and **choroid**.

transverse magnification
Magnification by making a larger image, e.g. **bright field magnifiers**. *Synonym is **real image magnification**.*

transverse plane
The anatomical plane that can be moved up and down the body. *Synonym is **axial plane**.*

TRD
Acronym of ***tractional retinal detachment.***

treponema pallidum
Bacteria that causes syphilis.

trichiasis
Ingrown **eyelash**es.

trichomegaly
Very long **eyelash**es.

trichotillomania
Behavioural disorder in which patients compulsively pull out hair. Commonly occurs to **eyelash**es and eyebrows, as well as the rest of the body.

trichromatism
Describes the condition of having (and being able to use) all three photopigments. Despite this, may have **anomalous trichromatism.**

trigeminal ganglion
Has three divisions: ophthalmic, maxillary, and mandibular.

trigeminal nerve
Cranial nerve V. Originates in the pons, and splits into three branches at the **trigeminal ganglion**. The ophthalmic division carries sensory information from the **cornea** and **conjunctiva**. *Synonym is* ***fifth cranial nerve.***

trigeminal spectacles
Very close-fitting spectacles, for patients with reduced facial and **corneal** sensitivity to avoid unintentional damage to the eyes.

trigemino-oculomotor synkinesis
Synonym of ***jaw winking.***

trisomy
Condition of having three copies of a chromosome in a nucleus.

tritan
Refers to **tritanope**s and **tritanomalope**s.

tritanomalope
An individual with a **tritanomaly**.

tritanomaly
Anomalous trichromatism in which more blue is required for colour matching. Very rare.

T

tritanope
An individual with **tritanopia**.

tritanopia
Dichromatism in which there is no **cyanolabe** pigment.

TRO
Acronym of ***tropicamide*****.**

trochlea
Pulley of cartilage attached to the **frontal bone**, through which the **superior oblique** passes.

trochlea fossa
Depression in the **frontal bone**, housing the **trochlea**.

trochlear nerve
Cranial nerve IV. Innervates the **contralateral superior oblique**. *Synonym is* ***fourth cranial nerve*****.**

troland
Candelas per square metre multiplied by the **pupil** area in square millimetres. *Abbreviation is* ***Td*****.**

tropia
Synonym of ***strabismus*****.**

tropicamide
An antimuscarinic **mydriatic**, routinely used by **optometrists**. Occasionally used as a **cycloplegic**. Typically available in 0.5% and 1% concentrations. *Acronym is* ***TRO*****.**

Troxler effect
The phenomenon seen after fixating on an area with no sharp edges for a time, in which peripheral perception disappears.

T

true distance exotropia
A **distance exotropia** due to **accommodation**.

Ts-cell
Abbreviation of suppressor T-cell.

TSA
Acronym of transverse spherical aberration.

Tscherning's ellipse
Used to estimate **Ostwalt forms** and **Wollaston forms** of **point focal lenses**.

TTS
*Acronym of **text-to-speech**.*

TTT
*Acronym of tear thinning time/**transpupillary thermotherapy**.*

tuberculosis
Infection by Mycobacterium tuberculosis. Can cause granulomatous **inflammation** of anterior and **posterior chamber.**

Tumbling E
An **optotype** chart comprising **Sloan letter** Es, each shown in one of four orientations.

tumour necrosis factor
Cytokine produced by macrophages that can cause apoptosis. *Acronym is **TNF**.*

tumour suppressor gene
Gene that reduces the chance that a cell will become a tumour.

tunica vasculosa lentis
Capillary network supplying the lens during foetal development. Disappears after birth.

Turville infinity balance
Septum placed on a mirror so that two sets of rings mounted on the wall are dissociated. *Acronym is **TIB**.*

twitch
A short muscle contraction.

two alternative forced choice method
Psychophysical test in which a stimulus is presented in one of two positions/time periods. Patient must choose between the two (so there are no confidence issues). *Acronym is **TAFC**.*

two position keratometer
A **keratometer** which measures each **corneal axis** separately. *Synonym is **fixed doubling keratometer**.*

two-channel theory
Theory of binocular vision which states that **rivalry** and **fusion** are two separate processes working in parallel.

Tx
Abbreviation of treatment.

tylosis
Thickening of the **eyelid** margin.

T

Tyndall effect
Any transparent medium of uniform **refractive index** appears optically empty, as no particles scatter light.

type 1 red-green colour vision defect
Similar to **protan** deficiency, associated with **macula**r pathology, loss of **visual acuity**, and central **visual field**.

type 2 red-green colour vision defect
Similar to **deutan** deficiency, associated with optic nerve pathology, loss of **visual acuity**, and central **visual field**.

type 3 tritan colour vision defect
Similar to **tritan** deficiency; luminous efficiency either reduced at both ends, or shifted down.

typoscope
Reading line guide **low vision** aid that makes it easier to track which line of text is being read.

tyrosinase
Enzyme involved in the production of melanin. **Albino** individuals may have some or none at all.

tyrosinase hair bulb test
Test for type of **albinism**: hair root is tested for presence of **tyrosinase**.

U

U
Abbreviation of use-only medicine.

U&S
Acronym of use-and-supply medicine.

Uhthoff phenomenon
The fact that vision worsens in patients with **optic neuritis** with body heat (e.g. during exercise).

ulcerative keratitis
*Synonym of **microbial infiltrative keratitis**.*

ultrasound scan
*Synonym of **echography**.*

uncrossed retinal disparity
Occurs behind the **horopter**. **Diplopia** occurs outside **Panum's fusional area**. *Synonyms are **homonymous retinal disparity**, **nasal retinal disparity**, and **negative retinal disparity**.*

underaccommodation
*Synonym of **accommodative lag**.*

unHARC
*Abbreviation of **unharmonious anomalous retinal correspondence**.*

unharmonious anomalous retinal correspondence
Anomalous retinal correspondence in which the patient is aware of a **strabismus**, but the magnitude is less than the objective angle of deviation. *Abbreviation is **unHARC**.*

unilateral
On one side.

unilateral neglect
Condition in which a patient has a full **visual field** but lacks the ability to pay attention to one **hemifield** (usually the left). There are three types: **egocentric unilateral neglect**, **allocentric unilateral neglect**, and **object-centred unilateral neglect**. *Synonyms are **hemifield neglect** and **hemispatial neglect**.*

Urrets-Zavalia syndrome
Condition occurring in a small group of keratoconics who, when given a **mydriatic**, remain dilated for weeks/months.

URTI
Acronym of upper respiratory tract infection.

Usher's syndrome
Inherited hearing impairment associated with **retinitis pigmentosa**.

USS
Acronym of ***ultrasound scan****.*

utrocular discrimination
Conscious awareness of which eye is viewing a stimulus. More common in individuals with binocular vision disorders.

UV
Acronym of ultraviolet.

uvea
The **choroid**, **ciliary body**, and iris. *Synonym is* ***uveal tract****.*

uveal tract
Synonym of ***uvea****.*

uveitis
Inflammation of any part of the **uvea**.

uveoscleral flow
One of the routes of **aqueous humour** drainage (~10%) into the supraciliary space, then veins and lymphatic vessels.

U

V

V
*Abbreviation of **constringence**/vision without correction.*

V number
*Synonym of **constringence**.*

V pattern
Increased **divergence** in **elevation** of ≥15 **prism dioptres**. Should be classified as **Veso** or **Vexo**.

V1
*Synonym of **primary visual cortex**.*

V2
Part of both the **magnocellular pathway** and **parvocellular pathway**, receiving information from **V1**. Contains **thin stripes**, **thick stripes**, and **interstripes**.

V3
Part of the **dorsal stream**, encoding motion. Receives input from **V2**.

V4
Part of the **ventral stream**, encoding colour, orientation, and spatial frequency. Receives input from **V2** and is tuned to stimuli of moderate complexity.

V5
*Synonym of **visual area middle temporal**.*

VA
*Acronym of **visual acuity**.*

van Herick's technique
Used to estimate the depth of the **anterior chamber**. Using a slit lamp, an optical section of light is shone at 60° next to the **limbus**. A comparison of the light width of the **corneal** section with the shadow between the corneal section and the iris is made.

vanishing optotype
A type of **visual acuity** test – target is an outlined area with the same overall brightness as the background. If the detail cannot be resolved, no target is seen.

variable doubling keratometer
*Synonym of **one position keratometer**.*

varicella-zoster virus
A virus that can go into hibernation and return again. Causes chickenpox at a young age. More serious at older age (shingles).

varices
Dilated veins.

vascular arcade
A group of arteries and veins.

vascular endothelial growth factor
Synonym of ***vascular endothelial growth factor-A****.*

vascular endothelial growth factor-A
A **cytokine** induced by **ischaemia**; causes **angiogenesis**; e.g. in diabetes and **wet age-related macular degeneration**. Previously known as 'vascular endothelial growth factor', but since then other variants have been discovered. *Synonym is* ***vascular endothelial growth factor****.*

vascularised limbal keratitis
Often caused by extended wear **rigid gas permeable** contact lenses. Extreme three and nine o'clock staining and limbal vessel encroachment.

vaso-obliteration
Stenosis due to thickening of vessel walls, e.g. cholesterol.

vasoproliferation
Continued growth of blood vessels (as opposed to **angiogenesis**).

Vcc
Acronym of vision with correction.

VDT
Acronym of visual display terminal.

VDU
Acronym of visual display unit.

VDW
Acronym of van der Waals.

V

VECP
Acronym of ***visual evoked cortical potential****.*

VECR
Acronym of ***visual evoked cortical response****.*

vection
A sense of self-motion due to **induced motion.**

VEGF
Acronym of ***vascular endothelial growth factor.***

veiling glare
Glare caused by a light that is so bright it can't be seen past.

veiling reflection
A reflection from a high luminance source that obscures the task, e.g. on a screen.

ventral
Anatomical term: front (of body, i.e. towards chest).

ventral stream
The 'what' of the visual system. Incorporates **V2, V4,** and the **inferotemporal cortex.**

VEP
Acronym of ***visual evoked potential.***

VER
Acronym of ***visual evoked response.***

vergence
The movement of both eyes in opposite directions. *Synonym is* ***disjunctive eye movement.***

vergence accommodation
Automatic **accommodation** stimulated by **convergence**. *Synonym is* ***convergence accommodation.***

Verhoeff membrane
A virtual membrane seen by **optical coherence tomography** between the **retinal pigment epithelium** and cone photoreceptors due to a change in **refractive index** at this point.

veridical
Truthful.

VERIS
Acronym of ***visual evoked response*** *imaging system.*

vernal keratoconjunctivitis
A form of **allergic conjunctivitis**. Bilateral. More common in males, and in the spring and summer. Causes cobblestone **papillae, Horner–Trantas dots**, papillary **hypertrophy**, and **shield ulcer**s. *Acronym is VKC.*

V

vernier acuity
A type of **localisation** acuity – the ability to judge whether two lines are separated or not.

version
Describes a binocular eye movement in which both eyes move in the same direction and by the same amount. *Synonym is* ***conjugate eye movement****.*

verteporfin
Protoxin used in **photodynamic therapy**. *Synonym is* ***Visudyne****.*

verteporfin photodynamic therapy
Synonym of ***photodynamic therapy****.*

vertex distance
Synonym of ***back vertex distance****.*

vertex power
Synonym of ***back vertex power****.*

vertex power allowance
Power allowance for a change in a lens's properties, often due to a change in **refractive index**.

vestibular gain
The amount of eye movement reflex in one direction in relation to the head movement in the opposite direction.

vestibular nerve
A division of the **vestibulocochlear nerve**. Innervated by the **kinocilia** of the **ampullae**. **Contralateral** projections are excitatory; **ipsilateral** projections are inhibitory.

vestibular nystagmus
Nystagmus associated with disorders of the vestibular system. Not to be confused with **vestibulo-ocular reflex nystagmus**.

vestibulo-ocular reflex
Eye movement driven by changes within the inner ear canal. Fast (~10 ms latency). Tested with the **Halmagyi–Curthoys head impulse test** and **caloric testing**. *Acronym is* ***VOR****.*

vestibulo-ocular reflex nystagmus
The reset phase that occurs when the far periphery of **gaze** is reached in the **vestibulo-ocular reflex**; e.g. when spinning around.

vestibulocochlear nerve
Cranial nerve VIII. Splits into two nerves: the **vestibular nerve** and the cochlear nerve.

VF
Acronym of ***visual field****.*

VFL
Acronym of ***visual field*** *loss.*

video magnifier
A **low vision aid** comprising a camera which the user directs at the object to be magnified, which is shown on a display. *Synonym is* ***CCTV magnifier.***

Vieth–Müller circle
Imaginary circle passing through the centre of rotation of each eye (once believed to be the **horopter**).

viewpoint invariance
The ability to recognise objects from a variety of angles, regardless of whether or not a given object has been seen from a given angle before.

VIP
Acronym of visually impaired patient.

viral conjunctivitis
Conjunctivitis with watery presentation, **follicles**, and swelling of the pre-auricular node.

Virchow's triad
Signs of **thrombosis**: injury to epithelia, slow blood flow, change of blood make-up.

virtual reality
Form of **extended reality** in which the user wears a **head-mounted display** which completely obscures the view of the real world.

Vis
Abbreviation of vision without correction.

visibility indicator
A printed **contrast** guide used by patients to work out how good their lighting is at home.

VISION 2020
An initiative by the World Health Organization which aimed to eliminate avoidable blindness by 2020.

visual acuity
A measure of the ability of an individual to resolve detail at high **contrast**. Can be expressed in many ways, often as a **Snellen fraction** or **logMAR** value. *Acronym is VA. Synonym is* ***acuity.***

visual agnosia
Inability to recognise objects despite having good vision. There are two types: **apperceptive visual agnosia** and **associative visual agnosia**. *Synonym is* ***agnosia.***

V

visual allesthesia
Perception of a visual image in the opposite **hemifield** to which it is presented. A form of **hallucination**.

visual anomia
Inability to name objects, despite not having **visual agnosia**. Due to damage between visual and language brain areas. *Synonym is **optic aphasia**.*

visual area medial superior temporal
Part of the **dorsal stream**; receives input from **visual area middle temporal**. Involved in motion processing and **optic flow**. *Acronym is MST. Synonym is **TO-2**.*

visual area middle temporal
Part of the **dorsal stream**, sensitive to movement. Projects to **visual area medial superior temporal**. Damage to this area causes **akinetopsia**. *Acronym is MT. Synonyms are **TO-1** and **V5**.*

visual association area
*Synonym of **extrastriate cortex**.*

visual association cortex
*Synonym of **extrastriate cortex**.*

visual attention span
In reading research, the number/spatial extent of letters that can be memorised from a brief presentation. Compare with **perceptual span** and **visual span**.

visual cortex
The **primary visual cortex** and the **extrastriate cortex** (areas **V2**, **V3**, **V4**, and **V5**). *Synonym is **occipital cortex**.*

visual evoked cortical potential
*Synonym of **visual evoked potential**.*

visual evoked cortical response
*Synonym of **visual evoked potential**.*

visual evoked potential
Measures signals evoked from the **visual cortex**. Primarily assesses the **macula** due to the effect of **cortical magnification**. *Acronym is VEP. Synonyms are **visual evoked cortical potential**, **visual evoked cortical response**, and **visual evoked response**.*

V

visual evoked response
*Synonym of **visual evoked potential**.*

visual extinction
Condition similar to **unilateral neglect**, in which stimuli in the **contralesional** hemifield are ignored only when presented at the same time as a stimulus in the **ipsilesional** hemifield.

visual field
Describes the full extent of area of vision that an eye can see. Defects in the visual field may cause gaps in vision. *Acronym is VF.*

visual field cut
A **scotoma** extending to the far periphery, as in **hemianopia**.

visual field indices
In some **perimetry** printouts, located at the bottom-right of the printout. Contains the **mean deviation**, **pattern standard deviation**, **short-term fluctuation**, and **corrected pattern standard deviation**.

visual imagery
Imagining or remembering visual percepts – despite no visual input, the **primary visual cortex** is still activated on **functional magnetic resonance imaging**.

visual impairment
*Synonym of **low vision**.*

visual lobe
*Synonym of **occipital lobe**.*

visual memory
Memory of visual percepts. Believed to be stored without high spatial frequencies.

visual migraine
*Synonym of **acephalgic migraine**.*

visual pigment
A chromophore and opsin. Joined by a Schiff base.

visual prosthesis
Implants in the **visual cortex** connected to digital cameras.

visual purple
*Synonym of **rhodopsin**.*

visual rehabilitation
Help to effectively use what vision remains and adapt to change in ability following vision loss.

visual span
In reading research, the number/spatial extent of letters that can be correctly read from a line of text without moving gaze. Compare with **perceptual span** and **visual attention span**.

visual stress
A cluster of symptoms experienced when viewing high-contrast patterns, typically around 3 cycles per degree. Includes blur, headaches, **asthenopia**, and illusory motion. *Synonyms are **Irlen syndrome, Meares–Irlen syndrome,** and **pattern glare**.*

Visudyne
*Synonym of **verteporfin**.*

visuscope
An **ophthalmoscope** with a graticule target for assessing **eccentric fixation**.

vitiligo
Patchy loss of skin pigment.

vitreal liquefaction
The natural process of the **vitreous humour** turning to liquid. Begins around four years of age, due to aggregation of collagen. Can eventually lead to a **posterior vitreous detachment**.

vitrectomy
Removal of a portion of the **vitreous humour**. Incision is made at the pars plana. Replaced by **saline** or silicone oil.

vitreolysis
Yttrium aluminium garnet laser used to destroy **floaters** in the **vitreous humour**.

vitreomacular traction
The adhered **vitreous** pulling on the **macula**.

vitreous
*Synonym of **vitreous humour**.*

vitreous detachment
*General form of **posterior vitreous detachment**.*

vitreous haemorrhage
*Synonym of **intragel haemorrhage**.*

vitreous humour
Gelatinous mass occupying the large chamber behind the lens. Comprises water, **hyaluronan**, chondroitin sulphate, **vitrican**, and heparan sulphate. Adheres to the **optic nerve head**, pars plana, **ora serrata**, **macula**, and some blood vessels. *Synonym is **vitreous**.*

vitreous prolapse
Condition in which the **vitreous humour** pokes into the **anterior chamber**; often after **cataract** surgery. Often a problem if rubbing the **corneal endothelium**.

vitrican
A constituent of **vitreous humour** that prevents aggregation of collagen.

VKC
Acronym of ***vernal keratoconjunctivitis***.

VKH
Acronym of ***Vogt–Koyanagi–Harada Syndrome***.

Vogt limbal girdle
Crescent line of white crystal opacities at the nasal/temporal **limbus**. Two types: **Vogt limbal girdle type I** and **Vogt limbal girdle type II**.

Vogt limbal girdle type I
Contains holes and has a clear perilimbal area similar to the **lucid interval of Vogt** in arcus.

Vogt limbal girdle type II
No holes or perilimbal clear area, seen in patients with renal failure on dialysis treatment.

Vogt–Koyanagi–Harada syndrome
Uveitis with meningitis, **poliosis**, and **vitiligo**. Can lead to a **serous retinal detachment**. *Acronym is* ***VKH***.

Vogt's striae
Fine white vertical striae in the **corneal stroma** or **Descemet's membrane**. Seen in **keratoconus**.

voluntary flutter
Synonym of ***voluntary nystagmus***.

voluntary nystagmus
The ability to produce a rapid, low amplitude, horizontal oscillation of the eyes during **accommodation** which is exhausted usually within a minute. 8% of the population are thought to have mastered the ability. *Synonyms are* ***hysterical flutter, hysterical nystagmus, ocular fibrillation, ocular shuddering, psychogenic flutter, psychological nystagmus, voluntary flutter, voluntary ocular fibrillation, voluntary ocular oscillation,*** *and* ***voluntary ocular tremor***.

voluntary ocular fibrillation
Synonym of ***voluntary nystagmus***.

voluntary ocular oscillation
Synonym of ***voluntary nystagmus***.

voluntary ocular tremor
Synonym of ***voluntary nystagmus***.

V

von Graefe sign
A lag of movement of the upper **eyelid** when looking down.

von Graefe test
The use of prism greater than a patient's **fusional reserve**s to displace one eye vertically. Horizontal prism is then introduced until the separated images align vertically (calculates horizontal deviation).

von Recklinghausen disease
Synonym of ***neurofibromatosis type 1.***

VOR
Acronym of ***vestibulo-ocular reflex.***

vortex keratopathy
Synonym of ***corneal verticillata.***

Vossius ring
A ring shaped pattern of pigment from the iris left on the lens epithelium following blunt trauma to the eye.

VPA
Acronym of ***vertex power allowance****/vertical palpebral aperture.*

VR
Acronym of ***virtual reality****/vitreoretinal.*

Vsc
Acronym of vision without correction.

V

W

Wallenberg syndrome
Synonym of ***lateral medullary syndrome.***

Wallerian degeneration
Degeneration of a nerve axon distal from the site of damage due to crushing.

Watzke–Allen test
The use of an indirect **ophthalmoscopy** lens to make a line beam that passes through the patient's **fovea**. The patient is asked if the line appears as a solid or broken line (which could indicate a **macular hole**).

wavefront-guided LASIK
LASIK which is more specific to the aberrometry of the **cornea**.

wavefront-optimised LASIK
Similar to **wavefront-guided LASIK** but attempts to maintain the same degree of **corneal** asphericity as before the treatment.

WBC
Acronym of white blood cell.

WC
Acronym of water content.

WD
Acronym of working distance.

Weber contrast
Contrast defined as the difference in luminance between the task and background, divided by the luminance of the background.

Weber's constant
Synonym of ***contrast threshold.***

Weber's law
The ratio between **increment threshold** and background intensity remains constant. In reference to vision, applies under **photopic** viewing conditions only. For **scotopic** viewing conditions, the **de Vries–Rose law** applies.

Weill–Marchesani syndrome
Rare condition causing high **myopia**, **microspherophakia**, **ectopia lentis**, and **glaucoma.**

Weiss ring
A faint white ring of glial tissue from the **optic nerve head**, due to previous **posterior vitreous detachment**.

Wernicke's encephalopathy
A syndrome that can cause upbeat **nystagmus**.

wet age-related macular degeneration
Age-related macular degeneration characterised by leakage from a **choroidal neovascular membrane**. Causes more severe and sudden visual loss than **dry age-related macular degeneration**. *Synonyms are **exudative age-related macular degeneration** and **neovascular age-related macular degeneration**.*

wet thyroid eye disease
Infiltrates move into the **extraocular muscle**s cause swelling of the muscles, which can reduce **motility**.

wettability
The property of a surface that takes into account the **wetting angle**. An important factor in contact lens design. A low wetting angle indicates high wettability.

wetting angle
The angle formed by moisture on a surface. Measured by **sessile drop method** or **captive bubble method**.

white with pressure
Pale areas of fundus that appear following **scleral indentation**. Occurs in around 35% of the population. *Acronym is **WWP**.*

white without pressure
Pale areas found in the peripheral **fundus** of around 30% of the population, often with a brown-red border. May look like a **retinal detachment**, and may increase risk of detachment. *Acronym is **WWOP**.*

Wieger's ligament
Circular attachment between the posterior lens and **vitreous humour**. *Synonym is **hyaloideocapsular ligament**.*

Wilbrand's knees
*Synonym of **knees of Wilbrand**.*

W

Wilson's disease
Inherited condition characterised by abnormal copper deposition in tissues. Causes **Kayser–Fleischer rings** and **sunflower cataract**s.

Wirt test
*Synonym of **Titmus test**.*

with-the-rule astigmatism
Astigmatism in which the negative **axis** is within 15° either side of horizontal (180°); the steepest meridian is vertical. *Acronym is **wtr**.*

Wolfring glands
*Synonym of **glands of Wolfring**.*

Wollaston form
A form of **point focal lens** with highest back surface power. Not really used very often.

Worth 4-dot
A test in which the patient views a diamond shape of dots: one white, one red, and two green. Assesses **simultaneous perception**.

Wratten 12b filter
A filter used in conjunction with a cobalt blue filter; eliminates blue reflected light to increase **contrast**.

wtr
*Acronym of **with-the-rule astigmatism**.*

WTT
Acronym of wearing time today.

WWOP
*Acronym of **white without pressure**.*

WWP
*Acronym of **white with pressure**.*

X

X
Abbreviation of ***exophoria****.*

X(T)
Abbreviation of intermittent ***exotropia****.*

xanthelasma
Synonym of ***xanthelasma palpebrarum****.*

xanthelasma palpebrarum
Cholesterol deposits in the skin, usually around the eyes. Indicates **hypercholesterolaemia**. *Plural is* ***xanthelasmata****. Synonym is* ***xanthelasma****.*

xanthelasmata
Plural of ***xanthelasma palpebrarum****.*

xanthophyll
A type of **carotenoid** present at the **macula**.

xanthopsia
Yellow **chromatopsia**.

xerophthalmia
Absolute failure of mucin secretion by the **goblet cells**, causing extreme dry eye.

xerosis
Synonym of ***xerosis cutis****.*

xerosis cutis
Dry skin. *Synonym is* ***xerosis****.*

XR
Acronym of ***extended reality****.*

XT
Abbreviation of ***exotropia****.*

Y

YAG
Acronym of ***yttrium aluminium garnet laser****.*

yaw
Describes a head turn in the left-right axis (shaking of the head in this axis would usually be interpreted as 'no').

yellow spot
Synonym of ***macula****.*

yo
Acronym of years old.

yoke muscle
Synonym of ***contralateral synergist****.*

Young–Helmholtz theory of colour
Theory that states that there are three cone types: **L-cones**, **M-cones**, and **S-cones**; each has a spectral sensitivity curve, and these curves overlap. This is the currently accepted theory of colour perception.

Young's modulus
Synonym of ***modulus of elasticity****.*

yttrium aluminium garnet laser
A laser used in iridotomy and **capsulotomy**. *Acronym is* ***YAG****.*

Z

ZATA
Acronym of zippy adaptive threshold algorithm.

ZCSBV
Acronym of ***zone of clear single binocular vision*****.**

zeaxanthin
A **xanthophyll** found in the **macula**.

Zeis glands
Accessory **sebaceous gland**s located in the **eyelash** follicles. *Synonym is* ***glands of Zeis*****.**

Zeiss four lens
An indirect goniolens that does not require coupling fluid. Has four mirrors.

Zeitraffer phenomenon
Perceptual disorder in which visual motion appears to be extremely rapid. Compare with **akinetopsia**.

zone of clear single binocular vision
The area on a **fusional reserves** graph in which vision is both clear and single. *Acronym is* ***ZCSBV*****.**

zonules of Zinn
Fibrous strands connecting the lens to the **ciliary body**. *Synonym is* ***suspensory ligaments*****.**

zonulysis
Nd:**yttrium aluminium garnet laser** is used to destroy the **zonules of Zinn** to completely dislocate a lens following **lens subluxation**.

zygomatic bone
Cheek bone; forms part of the **orbit**.

For Product Safety Concerns and Information please contact our EU
representative GPSR@taylorandfrancis.com
Taylor & Francis Verlag GmbH, Kaufingerstraße 24, 80331 München, Germany

www.ingramcontent.com/pod-product-compliance
Lightning Source LLC
LaVergne TN
LVHW020704050926
847199LV00060B/281
* 9 7 8 1 0 4 1 3 3 7 0 6 5 *